Melissa vs Fibromyalgia

My Journey Fighting Chronic Pain, Chronic Fatigue and Insomnia

Melissa Reynolds

This book is set in the Raleway and Linux Libertine fonts

Edited and formatted by Luke Parkes

Praise for
Melissa vs Fibromyalgia

"I wish this book had been around when I first got diagnosed."

—Deb, a Fibro Fighter

"This book is a very interesting read. It is packed full of information that is easy to understand and apply. The book reads quickly and doesn't weigh you down with heavy text. Melissa is a brilliant writer and I enjoy her work. I recommend her book if you have fibromyalgia or know someone who does."

—Jessie

"Another fine book by Melissa Reynolds. I like that every chapter is stand alone. You can start anywhere and go anywhere. You can read from back to front if you want."

—Danny van Leeuwen, Opa, RN, MPH, CPHQ

Health Hats (www.health-hats.com)

Praise for
Pregnancy & Fibromyalgia

"Lived experience + self-awareness + systems thinking + good storytelling is golden. Add brevity and it's priceless. Melissa's book is priceless."

—Danny van Leeuwen, Opa, RN, MPH, CPHQ

Health Hats (www.health-hats.com)

"Pregnancy and Fibromyalgia is a short, easy-to-digest run-down of things you can expect during a fibro pregnancy, and how to navigate them."

—Diane Murray

Spoonie Living (blog.spoonieliving.com)

"An invaluable resource for fibro baby mammas."

—Caz

Invisibly Me (www.invisiblyme.com)

Contents

Foreword

As I read through this again, my admiration for my sister has reached new heights. For a lot of her life, she has experienced so much with the Fibromyalgia, the Chronic Fatigue, and so on. Instead of giving up, she has managed to adjust her lifestyle in ways that work better for her.

Honestly, I am lucky to have her in my life; she has been one of my biggest role models for as long as I know. And I am glad that I have had the opportunity to learn so much about Fibromyalgia. Hopefully, you see what an amazingly strong, willful person she is as you read this book.

—Luke Parkes

Disclaimer

None of the content specified in this book is to be treated as medical advice and not as a replacement for a professional healthcare physician. I am not an expert in Fibromyalgia, Chronic Fatigue Syndrome or Myofascial Pain Syndrome; I am an expert in *my* experience. I share my experiences and research to help you be your own advocate and to make the experience of this illness more visible.

Introduction

"To know even one life has breathed easier
because you have lived. This is to have succeeded."

—Ralph Waldo Emerson

I write about my fight against chronic illness for two reasons. The first is as an outlet for myself. I don't have a lot of people who understand what I am fighting on a daily basis, and I have done a lot of this journey alone. The second is so that it may empower others to get on their journey to having a better wellbeing.

I am not a doctor or medical professional in any field. I am a person who has had to learn the hard way through nearly twenty years of fighting an illness that nobody believed existed. And I want to share what has helped me in case it helps you.

However, you should always check with your doctor before trying anything. I always check *www.drugs.com* for interactions when it comes to medicines and supplements before I bother taking the research to my doctor. Even if you don't have a doctor who is willing to help you, like I did for so long (and I pray so hard you have a great doctor who will partner with you in this fight), then you must research thoroughly before trying anything.

In most cases, things that have helped me are fairly benign in terms of side effects. *Go for a walk, walk a bit too far, have a pain flare up for a few days* kind of thing.

I use the term "Fibromyalgia" most often, as this is the only formal diagnosis I have. It was given to me by a GP who, when I took an article about Fibromyalgia to her, checked the tender points, knew my history, and basically said, "Sure, it is Fibromyalgia."

More recently, when I was referred to a rheumatologist, I asked if this was the correct diagnosis, but she didn't seem all that keen to give me the diagnosis. She referred me to the pain clinic, stating that she had no medicines that would help me.

However, the pain clinic specialists were a hit-and-miss. The first was fantastic and understanding and suggested I try two medications that I declined due to the level of potential side effects and lack of positive research around. The other was a miss – they dismissed me and suggested I look into sleep hygiene.

As you will see in this book, I employ a lot of the usual recommended sleep hygiene suggestions and I have researched and implemented a lot for myself.

I had suspected for a long time that my neck issues were separate from the Fibromyalgia, especially given that ibuprofen sometimes helped (where we are quite firmly told that these type of medicines don't help Fibromyalgia), and it felt quite different to the other pain.

In 2017, I finally met a physiotherapist who was studying myofascial pain syndrome and confirmed this is what was causing my neck issues – chronic, severe trigger points that only release by acupuncture needles being placed in them. When they get too tight, they will spasm, causing severe pain. They will also cause severe headaches, dizziness and nausea.

I have had to see a physiotherapist every two or three weeks for years to try to manage this one issue. The most recent issue to bother me, orthostatic intolerance, is more aligned with chronic fatigue syndrome (CFS), and I have come to realise that several of my symptoms fit the criteria for a CFS diagnosis.

I had also always suspected this as the fatigue came on suddenly during a severe bug that I contracted in my final semester of university. The illness held me captive for three weeks before I realised I needed to see a doctor. With antibiotics, it took a further three weeks to heal.

But the fatigue remained.

I have managed to make a dent in the fatigue with certain coping mechanisms, but the fatigue and the trigger points in my neck, back and shoulders are what bother me the most.

When I say "Fibromyalgia," it can be translated as "Fibromyalgia, CFS, myofascial pain syndrome and/or any other chronic illness that causes pain, fatigue, insomnia and brain fog."

In this book, I share my experience, what works for me, and things that I have learnt about health and life in general. Please let me know if this book helps you. Please let me know if there is something you do that I don't know about. I'd love to share the journey with you.

The Progression

My memory is a fickle creature. There appears to be no rhyme or reason as to why I remember some things but not others. Fatigue often interferes with it. There are some things that are burned into it. I remember the outline of the progression of the Fibromyalgia. I remember key events such as doctors who implied I was making my symptoms up. Why would a 17-year-old waste their time with specialists?

It started when I was 14 years old. I developed recurrent pain in my forearms that was diagnosed as tendonitis. I was sent on my way with a wrist support splint to use as needed. By 17, when I was at university, my shoulders would ache, and the burn would grow worse and worse until the end of the day when I would arrive home in tears.

About this time, the doctors sent me to a few specialists to see if they could figure out what was going on. After several appointments and tests, one doctor basically implied I was making it up, because the pain changed. Some days, it was there; others, it wasn't. The intensity also changed.

So I carried on alone. Just pushing through the pain.

At 21, in my last semester of university, I came down with a terrible bug. It was like a super-charged cold. The fatigue was out of this world. I recall 9am tutorials in Romanticism (my favourite paper in my English Literature major) where I could barely hold my eyes open. Matchsticks seemed like the only option. At the time, I was attempting to work at a bagel shop; one shift required two bottles of V energy drink to get through.

After three weeks of absolute struggle, I went to the doctor. They never told me what it was, but they gave me antibiotics and told me to rest. It took three more weeks to clear.

But the fatigue never lifted.

It receded a little, but from that time onwards, chronic fatigue was a factor in my life, along with the growing chronic pain.

Sometime after this, I happened to see a locum who put me on amitriptyline due to my chronic insomnia. He never said why he suggested it, or if he wondered if I had Fibromyalgia. I hadn't heard of it yet.

After this, a friend who was living in the UK at the time sent me an article. This article put me on the beginning of my long journey toward wellness. It talked about Fibromyalgia as an explanation for the chronic pain, fatigue, and insomnia I suffered from.

My general practitioner heard me out, checked my tender points, and agreed I had Fibromyalgia – and then that was it.

She did nothing else.

So I was still on my own, but with a word that no one seemed to know about. This was before there were books in our libraries about Fibromyalgia or research freely available on the internet. But I was too sick to even think about researching for myself.

With my first full-time job came the neck and back progression. Being at the computer from 8.30am to 5.30pm did not help. Neither did the 1.5 hour commute each way.

At that time, I began to see a chiropractor, who really didn't help at all. After this, I tried massage therapy, which helped very little. Each week, I would look forward to my appointment, imbuing it with potential magical powers for making me feel better. Each week, I was disappointed.

At 25, I was working 9am to 5pm at a non-profit organisation and seeing a physiotherapist who did dry needling. She would essentially prod certain muscles in my shoulders and neck with a needle to make them jump (and hopefully, release).

Each day, I crawled out of bed at 5am, heated my heat pack, and lay in bed letting the warmth infuse movement back into my neck. Feeling so sore that it made me nauseous, I would make it into work, with a coffee to keep me awake and then a pain killer to make my body work. This would make my stomach very sore.

From about 3pm, I would struggle to keep my eyes open and cope with the pain. The 3-5pm block was the worst. Then I spent the entire one-hour bus ride home trying not to vomit, cry, or pass out.

I was miserable.

I genuinely wondered how I kept going.

I had this idea that if I could work slightly less, then my pain might reduce a little, too. It might make life more bearable. So, when my parents asked me to move with them to Auckland (a warmer city at the top of New Zealand), I agreed eagerly.

And that is when the better part of my story begins.

What is Fibromyalgia, Chronic Fatigue Syndrome and Myofascial Pain Syndrome?

Fibromyalgia is a chronic pain-based illness of unknown origin and cure. It affects approximately 3-6% of the world's population. It is said to occur far more often in women than men. It appears to be blind to race, education level and socioeconomic demographics. On the University of Maryland Medical Center website, it is explained in this way:

"Fibromyalgia is a chronic condition characterized by pain in the muscles, ligaments, and tendons; fatigue; and multiple tender points on the body."

And on the same page, they list the signs and symptoms of Fibromyalgia:

Widespread pain and stiffness   *Headaches*
Fatigue [and]/or trouble   *Pain after exertion*
sleeping   *Memory lapses/difficulty*
Paresthesia (tingling)   *concentrating*
Irritable bowel syndrome (IBS)   *Restless leg syndrome (RLS)*

Skin sensitivity	*Dizziness*
Heightened sensitivity to	*Anxiety*
noises, bright lights, smells	*Hemorrhoids*
Depression	

However, the trouble is that Fibromyalgia seems to be very unique to each person: how it comes on, what symptoms are present, what helps said symptoms. There is also a debate as to whether trigger points are present in Fibromyalgia or part of a separate issue called Myofascial Pain Syndrome. A lot of the above symptoms overlap with a lot of different conditions.

Some Associated Physiological Abnormalities

Research has found alterations in neurotransmitter regulation, immune system function, sleep physiology and hormone level control. A lot of research suggests that Fibromyalgia is the result of central nervous system dysfunction – specifically an overactive nervous system, stressing and exhausting the brain (Dennis W. Dobritt, *Fibromyalgia – A Brief Overview*).

Diagnosis

There are not many fibromyalgia fighters who have a short diagnosis story. A study of 800 patients found it took an average of 2.3 years and seeing 3.7 doctors prior to receiving a diagnosis[1]. It took me several years as the symptoms came on slowly and I was young; the doctors were disinclined to believe me, especially as my symptoms and their severity changed.

It is a tricky diagnosis: Fibromyalgia is often referred to as a "wastebasket" diagnosis. Doctors do have to rule out other illnesses before they can diagnose it. There is no specific test for Fibromyalgia that is widely used yet. The symptoms are generalised: widespread pain on both sides of the body (subjective) for at least three months, fatigue, difficulty sleeping and difficulty concentrating.

The tender point count used to be one of the defining features of diagnosis. However, tender points were found to be unreliable; you needed 11 of 18 to be diagnosed, and some days, you could have at least that many; others, you may

---

[1] Ernest Choy et al. 2010. A patient survey of the impact of fibromyalgia and the journey to diagnosis. Retrieved from https://www.ncbi.nlm.nih.gov/pmc/articles/PMC2874550/

have less. Often, you also have to find a doctor who wants to help you and believes in Fibromyalgia. I do so hope this is becoming a thing of the past, but it certainly was an issue for me.

The medical profession doesn't seem clear yet on whether it is a central nervous system disorder, immune based, neurological, or all of the above. What has been made clear in the last few decades of research is that it is *not* psychosomatic. However, it is an illness with physiological effects, despite most of the symptoms being invisible.

Misdiagnosis

One issue with Fibromyalgia, besides the difficulty in obtaining a diagnosis and help, is misdiagnosis. One research paper (Fitzcharles & Boulos, *Inaccuracy in the diagnosis of fibromyalgia syndrome*) puts it this way:

> *"There is a disturbing inaccuracy, mostly observed to be over diagnosis, in the diagnosis of FM by referring physicians. This finding may help explain the current high reported rates of FM and caution*

physicians to consider other diagnostic possibilities when addressing diffuse musculoskeletal pain."

One doctor who writes about Fibromyalgia, David Brady, posits that as many as two thirds of patients may be misdiagnosed. Interestingly, one of the things that he finds often misdiagnosed as "classic Fibromyalgia" is Myofascial Pain Syndrome, whereas in my case, there is the presence of both – which adds another layer of complexity to these illnesses. Other issues misattributed to Fibromyalgia include thyroid problems, Lyme disease and nutritional deficiencies, as well as other illnesses.

For an interview with him about misdiagnosis see this blog post[2] from Fed up with Fatigue.

History

Fibromyalgia is not a new illness. There is mention of it under other names going back centuries. In her article *The History of Fibromyalgia* (2017) (on *verywell.com*), Adrienne Dellwo writes:

---

[2] Physician says fibromyalgia misdiagnosis is rampant. 2017. Retrieved from https://fedupwithfatigue.com/fibromyalgia-misdiagnosis/

*"In 1592, French physician Guillaume de Baillou intro-
duced the term 'rheumatism' to describe musculoskeletal pain that didn't originate from injury. This was
a broad term that would have included fibromyalgia
as well as arthritis and many other illnesses."*

And in the journal article *History of Fibromyalgia* (2004)
(available on the PubMed website), the authors, Inanici and
Yunus, say this:

*"For several centuries, muscle pains have been
known as rheumatism and then as muscular rheumatism. The term fibrositis was coined by Gowers
in 1904 and was not changed to fibromyalgia until
1976. Smythe laid the foundation of modern FMS in
1972 by describing widespread pain and tender
points."*

What is so disconcerting is that, despite hundreds of
years of doctors documenting people suffering from this illness – and my suffering right in front of their faces – people
refuse to believe it. I have been considered lazy and told I

ought to "push through," the difficulties of fighting this illness outright ignored.

I am trying to learn to get by without understanding or support, but with the information in this section, I hope that anyone suffering from this illness knows they are not alone. There is a long history.

There are many people fighting this with you – an estimated 3-6% worldwide[3] – and there are a boatload of amazing writers who share their journey as I am doing here.

Chronic Fatigue Syndrome

There doesn't yet seem to be an agreement as to whether Chronic Fatigue Syndrome (CFS) is on the other side of a spectrum from Fibromyalgia, where pain is the most prominent on the Fibromyalgia side and fatigue is the most prominent on the CFS side, or if CFS is a distinct illness. There are a lot of overlapping symptoms.

The key symptoms of CFS are:

- Extreme fatigue, persisting despite rest, for more than six months

---

[3] National Fibromyalgia & Chronic Pain Association. (n.d.). Prevalence. NFMCPA. Retrieved from the website https://www.fmcpaware.org/fibromyalgia/prevalence.html

- Post exertional malaise
- Sleep problems
- Pain
- Cognitive impairment
- Orthostatic intolerance

I have experienced many of these. Perhaps the most significant – besides the fatigue and pain – are the cognitive symptoms. Losing words, swapping words and short-term memory loss are all very disruptive to life, and especially work life.

Orthostatic intolerance – which, for me, manifests in the form of being dizzy for a few minutes if I stand up too fast as a result of my blood pressure dropping – can be mild or more debilitating. When I'm more fatigued or unwell, the dizziness can be so profound that I feel like I'm going to faint.

On the *Arthritis Foundation* website, Dr John Klippel, MD, discusses the differences and similarities of Chronic Fatigue Syndrome and Fibromyalgia and concludes that the treatment for either illness is similar.

On his website *EndFatigue*, Dr Jacob Teitelbaum, MD, calls Fibromyalgia a "sister illness" to CFS, and his treatment protocol is laid out in detail. His book *From Fatigued to Fantastic* (2007) refers to both together: "CFS/FM." The page on his website discussing his protocol and the research also refers to Myofascial Pain Syndrome.

Myofascial Pain Syndrome

Myofascial Pain Syndrome (MPS) is a chronic, painful condition that involves specific trigger points. The pain can be local or referred. A good definition of MPS that I have come across explains that it is: "hyperirritable spots, usually within a taut band of skeletal muscle or in the muscle's fascia that is painful on compression and can give rise to characteristic referred pain, tenderness, and autonomic phenomena"[4].

Signs and symptoms may include:

- Deep, aching pain in a muscle
- Pain that persists or worsens
- A tender knot in a muscle
- Difficulty sleeping due to pain[5]

There is often confusion between the tender points characteristic of Fibromyalgia and trigger points. The propensity

---

[4] Travell. JG, Simons, DG. Myofascial Pain and Dysfunction. The Trigger Point Manual: Upper Half of Body, 2nd edition. Lippincott, Williams & Wilkins, Baltimore 1988

[5] Mayo Clinic. (n.d.) *Myofascial Pain Syndrome*. Mayo Clinic. Retrieved from the website mayoclinic.org

for medical professionals to throw every symptom into the Fibromyalgia basket set me back for a decade. If they had realised prior to 2017 that my neck pain was really caused by trigger points, then we could have begun working on them sooner. These tiny hyperirritable spots have caused me over ten years of sleepless nights and 24/7 pain that nothing completely relieved.

MPS does not have universally accepted diagnostic criteria, so it also does not have reliable statistics as to the prevalence. An estimate, using data around musculoskeletal pain in general puts estimates of myofascial pain as a patient's primary complaint at 30%.[6]

The above literature review discusses general treatments for MPS: aside from eliminating as many aggravators of the condition as possible (like proper ergonomic posture at computers), treating any other present diseases, the treatment usually includes NSAIDS (usually stated as unhelpful for Fibromyalgia), heat pack, and acupuncture applied by a specific methodology.

---

[6] Overview of soft tissue rheumatic disorders .Irving Kushner, MDSection Editor:Zacharia Isaac, MDDeputy Editor:Monica Ramirez Curtis, MD, MPH Literature review current through: Mar 2018.. Last updated: May 12, 2017. on UptoDate.com.

Some research suggests MPS may develop into Fibromyalgia (see Mayo Clinic). In my experience, the Fibromyalgia came first, and then the central sensitivity opened the way for the myofascial pain.

How I Look at Them

Most of my coping mechanisms are whole of life (for me as a human being, for Fibromyalgia, CFS, and MPS); I look at my body as a whole and try to set good foundations, which, in turn, positively impacts the symptoms I experience.

There are differing treatments for certain symptoms. For example, I need a specific treatment for my neck and upper back (MPS) in order to function. This is different to the way I manage the wider spread pain by taking amitriptyline, reducing activity levels, and then managing the pain as it occurs.

I have only begun to tease the separate strands out, in case there is something I can try to help niggling symptoms.

Healing Journey Continued

It has taken me many years, thousands of dollars on treatments, reams of paper worth of research, and a lot of hard work to get this far on my wellness journey. I will not stop fighting. I believe I will always need to exert a little more energy than most people to manage my health – and that is alright.

Something I am working on is trying to accept my position as adjacent to "normal." I may look and sound "normal," but my energy levels and pain levels hold me back. Unfortunately, they are invisible, so unless people care to look deeper, they'll never understand.

I have gone from struggling every single day, wondering how I didn't pass out from the pain and fatigue I was feeling, to mostly functioning. And I am profoundly grateful. I didn't want to keep living like that. I will never let myself get back to that.

But it is difficult to accept this box I live in – the carefully constructed walls that enable me to achieve what I do. It is a balance between pain levels and functionality. I have to constantly remind myself that I have boundaries and limits for good reason. It all starts with me claiming the fact that I don't deserve to live in misery. That I can change my life. That it's my responsibility to be as well as I can. I cannot be a good mama or wife if I have not first looked after myself. In a culture of go-go-go living with four high-energy boys, it can be difficult to justify rest, time alone, and all of my self-care mechanisms. However, it takes a long time to build back up if I let it all fall down.

It took nearly 20 years coping with the symptoms of this illness, three pregnancies and first years (the most draining time of a person's life) to realise that I can continually push myself. I can dredge through and continue to live with high levels of pain at great cost to my quality of life. But if I fight for it, I can also reduce my pain.

For a long time, I prided myself on being a 60 on the CFS/Fibromyalgia Rating Scale[7], which states:

---

* My Italics

[7] CFIDS & Fibromyalgia Self-Help. (n.d.). *CFS & Fibromyalgia Rating Scale.* CFIDS & Fibromyalgia Self-Help. Retrieved from the website http://www.cfidsselfhelp.org

"Able to do about 6-7 hours of work a day.
Mostly mild to moderate symptoms" (despite pain
levels more in line with a 50) "able to do 4-5 hours
a day of work or similar activity at home. *Daily
rest required. Symptoms mostly moderate*.*"

I pushed myself to 6-7 hours per day minimum and suffered moderate symptoms. I had missed the key as suggested in this article on understanding our situation: "What is the highest level of functioning I can sustain *without intensifying** my symptoms?"[8]. If my pain is at a moderate level, then I should not be striving to work the hours of a person with more mild symptoms, especially given that I go home to small children as opposed to being able to rest. You need to take into account your symptom level and your situation.

I keep myself in the boom-bust pain-fatigue cycle. Well, me and my circumstances – I have small children and our financial hygiene dictates that I need to work at least part-time. I must learn to balance all of these demands. And that is going to be my life's work – balancing life with the fight against these illnesses.

---

* My Italics

[8] Bruce Campbell. (n.d.). *Understanding Your Situation*. CFIDS & Fibromyalgia Self-Help. Retrieved from the website http://www.cfidsselfhelp.org/

The 2018 Mindset Shift

The Fibromyalgia Grid

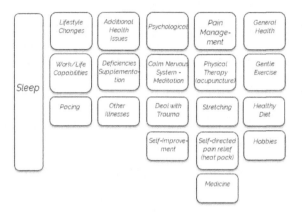

Once I finally started getting sleep thanks to low dose naltrexone, I realised that my premise that sleep was the missing key for me was correct. All those doctors writing specifically about treating Fibromyalgia, especially the ones that have it themselves, are right. You can still make a lot of progress by doing the many things I was doing, but you can't truly impact your quality of life until you sleep.

Temporarily, do whatever you need to do to get your sleep. I will talk about this in the sleep chapter with the research to back it up.

As I began to sleep in blocks of more than one hour at a time (presumably completing sleep cycles), I felt other benefits. Namely a reduction in fatigue, an increase in stamina and a decrease in pain. This had a very positive effect emotionally too.

Thankfully I had already been pursuing many of the strands that needed to be targeted. I knew that I needed to be following the general health rules for wellbeing such as eating healthily and exercising as I could. I had also been meditating for years, it was purely for rest purposes, but the other side effect was a calming of my central nervous system.

My doctor had helped me to keep an eye on nutritional deficiencies and we became aggressive when my iron levels dropped (injections rather than trying the supplements, which we knew didn't work).

Addressing the myofascial pain syndrome was tremendously helpful, as a lot of my pain stems from these nasty trigger points.

One thing that I had slowly been realising is that I had some past trauma to look into as it was definitely feeding into my current reactions.

I cannot say if full recovery is possible, but I wholly believe that we have the power to impact our quality of life. My quality of life has improved in such a manner that I am hopeful for more improvement once my children are no longer reliant upon me in the middle of the night or upon my body physically.

First Steps: The Order I Would Tackle Things In

When you are first diagnosed with a chronic illness such as Fibromyalgia or Chronic Fatigue Syndrome, your brain has rather a lot to process. If you're buried too deep in pain and fatigue, the enormity of the challenge may not hit you immediately. You, like me, may have been diagnosed after a long battle in which you have learnt to push through and assimilate the challenges into your life. Potentially making yourself even worse. Or you may have been struck down, as if by a lightning bolt of pain and fatigue.

Here is what I would do if I started over:

Research

You are your advocate, medical coordinator, cheerleader and guru. You need to guide your doctor. You need to track your progress. Get a book or open a digital file and write it up. Keep articles that you come across. Because when you're ready, you need to experiment. But your doctor can only take you so far. I highly recommend reading *From Fatigued to Fantastic* (2001) by Dr Jacob Teitelbaum and *The FibroManual: A Complete Treatment Guide to Fibromyalgia for You and Your Doctor* (2016) by Dr Ginevra Liptan. These two authors are doctors who have fibromyalgia themselves. Their processes are useful and a good place to start.

Prioritise Sleep

However you need to get it, do it. I have written several posts on this on my blog and have a chapter in this book on sleep. I really hope your doctor recognises the importance of sleep in the body's ability to function. You need to do everything in your power to get enough sleep in order to be well.

Do the Work

There are many types of treatments, medicines, supplements, alternative treatments, physical treatments, and diets. We all have different chemical make ups, different genetics, and different triggers. This means we need to find our lifestyle that gets us as pain free and awake as possible.

The complexity of this is huge, especially when you take in the fact that synergies, mixtures of things, may be the solution. Your body may need a mixture of medicines, supplements, physical work and mental work.

Hit Your Lifestyle

You can't keep going in the same way. That way didn't work. Try to journal it out or talk it out, or whatever you do to think things through. You need to rebuild your lifestyle. Find what works for you, what your passions are (the non-negotiables of your life) and go from there. I spent a long time dreaming of working slightly less hours so that I could rest more and try to recover.

Find Your People

If there's no one in real life, find a virtual community. You need to be exposed to new ideas and you need to be able to ask questions. There are many people struggling along with chronic illnesses sharing their journey. Just try to keep it positive. Most people would have brushes with depression/sadness when they're in daily pain and exhaustion.

Start Meditating/Working on Your Central Nervous System

At first meditation was solely for deep rest where none could be obtained any other way. But it's made a huge difference in a great many ways, as I discuss in the chapter on meditation. An emerging theme of treatments popping up is calming the central nervous system and reducing the heightened fight or flight response, often prevalent in Fibromyalgia fighters.

Summary

This would be the core list of things to start with, but really, this entire book could be entitled as this chapter is. This book is all the things I've done that help me. There are so many more options and ideas out there so long as you're able keep your eyes and ears open.

What I do: Sleep

Sleep is the cornerstone, the foundation upon which everything else is built. I've tried all the supplements, all the exercises, stretches, ate well, and experimented a lot, but full wellbeing is impossible without sleep.

I feel like the sleep disorder part of Fibromyalgia is really overlooked. It certainly has been in my experience with the New Zealand medical system. Sleep is a basic human necessity. Yet we live in chronic sleep deprivation.

Sleep Research

Dr Ginevra Liptan, MD, writes about this in her book *The Fibro Manual* (2016):

> "*Sleep studies show that Fibromyalgia subjects show abnormal 'awake-type' brain waves all night long, with reduced and interrupted deep sleep and frequent 'mini-awakenings' (Brandi 1994; Kooh 2003). This deep-sleep deprivation leads to pain, fatigue, and poor brain function (Lerma 2011; Moldofsky 2008; Harding 1998). Treatment focused on*

increasing deep sleep is the key to improving all these symptoms."

In plain terms, people with Fibromyalgia don't tend to reach stage four of the sleep cycle (the deep, restorative stage), and therefore, they suffer from chronic, deep sleep deprivation, which causes all sorts of issues with the body: pain, fatigue, fog, anxiety, etc.

In his article, *8 Tips for Better, More Effective Sleep* (n.d.) (available on the Paleohacks website), Casey Thaler explains that sleep deprivation is "very similar to speeding up the process of dying of old age." No wonder we feel like Fibromyalgia is progressive – our bodies are progressing toward death until we take the sleep problem seriously.

The research on sleep is fascinating, and I learnt a lot reading *Night School: Wake up to the Power of Sleep* by Richard Wiseman.

What is interesting is that I appear to follow the usual circadian rhythm, my body will start waking up at 7am, peak at 11am, decline to the lowest point by 3, climb and peak again around 7 with my body seeking sleep from 9. So I assume I just have slightly weaker ability to wake and sleep than others, while still following the natural pattern.

Wiseman references a lot of research. For example, in 2006 it was "estimated that around sixty million Americans suffer from a chronic sleep disorder" (p57) and approximately a third of Americans now get less than seven hours of sleep per night. In a British study more than 30% of participants had insomnia or another serious sleep problem. With this setting the scene, Wiseman goes on to explain what happens when you don't get enough sleep – spoiler alert, nothing good.

"Belenskys's study reveals the highly pernicious nature of even a small amount of sleep deprivation. Just a few nights sleeping for seven hours or less and your brain goes into slow motion. To make matters worse you will continue to feel fine and so don't make allowances for your sluggish mind. Within just a couple of days this level of sleep deprivation transforms you into an accident waiting to happen." (P67)

In a talk in 2013 Dr Jacob Teitelbaum said the defining way to separate Fibromyalgia from any other cause of widespread pain and fatigue is to ask how well they sleep. If a patient sleeps with no trouble, according to Teitelbaum, they don't have Fibromyalgia. His SHINE protocol puts sleep at the beginning of the treatment. Without sleep, we can't get better. I would agree. Both of Teitelbaum's books have resonated with me and his treatment approach gels with everything I have experienced. Without the sleep LDN was able to give me, I would never have begun to experience the rest of the improvements. Though I do wonder, of the large percentages of people in his studies that are lots better or better after the SHINE protocol, what that "better" means for them. For me, my quality of life is currently hugely improved, but I still definitely have a chronic illness that impacts me all day, every day. We might have different definitions of improvement.

Taking Sleep Seriously

Does anyone else find it ridiculous that many millions of people are exhausted; struggle to get to sleep, to stay asleep, to wake feeling refreshed, to have sufficient energy to live; yet their doctors are not (generally) working their butts off to help find a solution?

After ten years battling Fibromyalgia mostly alone, I was referred to a pain specialist at the hospital, and she dismissed my sleep problems, saying medicine won't help and I should try some more sleep hygiene. Now, I go to bed around the same time every day, don't have caffeine after lunch, take my time to wind down, do a body scan meditation before going to sleep, partake in gentle exercise most days, and so on. I have also tried chamomile tea, Sleep Drops, 5-HTP, melatonin, and magnesium, and I have been on amitriptyline for around ten years. I have done all of these things for a long time. I wouldn't have been begging for help or looking into medicine if anything had worked.

I have always known that sleep makes a massive difference for me. If I can spend nine hours in bed to achieve eight hours of broken sleep, I feel so much better.

FUN FACT

On the website Talk About Sleep, *Fibromyalgia is located under "sleep disorders."*

Dr Jacob Teitelbaum, MD, and Dr Genevra Liptan, MD, are two prominent physicians who have Fibromyalgia and write about how to recover – and sleep is the basis for recovery. They recommend both natural and pharmaceutical options, and they acknowledge how important sleep is to getting well.

I have come a long way. I have implemented an entire lifestyle change including reduced work hours, supplementation, gentle exercise, meditation and rest. But I couldn't get any further without help with my sleep.

This is where Low Dose Naltrexone (LDN) came in. You can learn more about LDN in the chapter dedicated to it. Essentially this medicine finally helped me to sleep in more than one hour blocks. The flow on effect of this has improved the quality of my life dramatically. Not fighting so hard for sleep, achieving sleep cycles and getting proper sleep has made as big a difference as I hypothesized it would.

Based upon the estimate that Dr David Hanscom mentions in his book *Back in Control: A Surgeon's Journey Out of Chronic Pain* of 40% of those with insomnia developing chronic pain and my experience, my number one recommendation to anyone suffering from chronic pain or similar illnesses is to get your sleep.

Things That Can Help

Sleep hygiene is something you will probably hear about at some point. It is a set of tips that can make getting to sleep easier. There are a lot of options, so you have to create a sleep hygiene routine that works for you.

Here are some basic sleep hygiene tips that I follow:

- Don't have caffeine after lunch.
- Have a wind-down routine (that doesn't involve technology!).
- Go to bed and get up at approximately the same time each day.
- Expose yourself to sunlight early in the day.
- Adjust your bed to your needs (i.e. suitable mattress, mattress topper, the right pillow, weather-suitable blankets).
- Eat a small protein-based snack before bed.
- Have a warm bath with Epsom salts.
- Apply magnesium oil.
- Manage the pain as best as you can.
- Dab lavender oil on temples and wrists.
- Use your heat pack (I heat it up right before bed and go to sleep with it behind my neck/shoulders).
- Do a body scan meditation (I do one right before I go to sleep and again if I wake in the night).

Here are some natural sleep aids you can try:

- Revitalizing Sleep Formula (an all in one herbal mix).
- Other formulas with the herbal sleep remedies such as Valerian root.
- Lemon balm
- GABA supplement
- Chamomile tea
- 5-HTP
- Essential oils
- Melatonin

Other sleep helps:

- Amitriptyline or other prescribed antidepressant (I took it for over a decade and finally was able to come off it once the LDN was helping.)
- Over the counter medicines to help with sleep.
- Pain relief (a part of my sleep woes are due to neck pain, prior to bed I take a dose of pain medicine, if needed, to help get a jump start on the night);

- Temporary use of prescribed sleep aids as prescribed and monitored by your doctor.

You may find the template on the next page useful for tracking your sleep and any sleep hygiene methods you enact (it is available to download on my website).

Sleep Diary		
Date	Hours	Supplements/Medicines

What I do: Pain Relief

This chapter would have looked differently if I had written it prior to 2017. I seem to have gathered the right strands together to create the best pain relief plan possible. This book is a love song to all the things I do that help. This chapter will focus on all the ways I know to ease pain.

You can't control pain well without first reducing what causes or amplifies the pain. There is no point popping pills if you are not taking care of yourself. Most of the things I do to be well are basic healthy living guidelines.

Please don't be daunted by all the things I do – it is an exhaustive list because not everything works for everyone; it is my hope there is something here that helps you.

My Specific Regimen
Lifestyle focused

- Sleep effects pain levels like nobody's business. I have a comprehensive sleep hygiene plan that I follow and this includes medicine. (For more, see the chapter on sleep.)

- Keep moving even when it seems near impossible. Refer to the chapter *What I do: Gentle Exercise.*

- Incorporating rest into the day is necessary. Regular periods of rest with my heat pack reduce the amount of pain at bedtime, making it easier to get to sleep. A 20-30 minute meditation is more refreshing than attempting to nap (I am a terrible napper), and it is one of the best tools I have in my arsenal.

- Try to see food as fuel and, therefore, nourish myself appropriately.

- I only work part-time. Prior to children, that was ¾ time and now it is half time.

Specific For Pain

- I take low dose naltrexone (LDN) about 9pm in the evening. Over a period of a year, it decreased my neck pain levels more than anything ever has (likely due to helping me sleep). It is not a miracle drug – if I don't take it, the fatigue skyrockets, and if I overdo it, my neck pain increases. It is part of a whole lifestyle plan for wellness, the thing that made this chapter different than before. (For more information, see the chapter about it.)

- For a long time, the only thing I had was a low dose of amitriptyline. It would help me get to sleep where nothing else has ever worked, it also helped with some of the wide spread pain.

- My heat pack is my first line of defence. I use it on my neck first thing, whenever I can during the day, in the evening and at bedtime.

- If I can't use my heat pack or I cannot sit around with it, I will use Deep Heat, a non-medicated heat producing rub that eases muscle pain, especially when combined with a good massage.

- A hot bath is my best treat and the first thing I want when the pain increases.

- MSM (Methylsulfonylmethane) for muscle and joint pain. It helped with the pain in my index fingers during the coldest months as well as a little difference in my neck.

- Slow release, high dose ibuprofen for period pain, for about four days – it's pretty severe.

- Ibuprofen or paracetamol (Acetaminophen) for headaches or low level pain.

- A muscle relaxant for spasms in the neck or back – the frequency of these has decreased since I began LDN.

- I see the physiotherapist every two or three weeks and they do neck tractions/mobilisations and place acupuncture needles in trigger points in my neck and shoulders. This is the only thing that keeps the neck free and keeps the severe headaches, dizziness and nausea that accompanies the severe neck pain.
- A theracane trigger point massager for self-trigger point release.
- I apply magnesium oil to my back and shoulders at bedtime.

Some Natural Pain Relief Methods

- Heat pack
- Ice pack
- Hot bath or shower (bonus add some lavender and/or chamomile essential oils)
- For a bad headache: feet in hot water, ice pack around neck
- For headaches or muscle tension: Peppermint oil with a carrier oil (I always have coconut oil on hand and it's less greasy than others) on the temples.

- Lavender oil massaged into your feet or neck/temples if you can handle the smell
- Check all nutrient levels and supplement where needed – especially magnesium and iron.
- Meditation. Look up "Guided Mindfulness Meditation on Coping with Pain (20 Minutes)" on YouTube.
- Homeopathic remedies
- Yoga routines for chronic illness (see the Yoga chapter for more information)
- Cat and cow pose
- Self-trigger-point work
    - Acupressure release
    - Theracane trigger point massager
    - Foam roller
- Rest and sleep – get as much as possible
- Physiotherapy with acupuncture – especially for trigger points.
- Teas/Infusions with potential benefits
    - Turmeric
    - Thyme
    - Chamomile
    - Nettle
    - Red Raspberry Leaf

- Supplements
  - MSM
  - Curcumin
  - Energy Revitalisation Formula
  - FibroMalic (Malic acid)
  - Magnesium
  - Fish oil
  - Acetyl L-carnitine
  - 5-HTP (not to be taken with some medications such as antidepressants)
  - SAMe (not to be taken with some medications such as antidepressants)
- Massage: self-massage, partner/friend massage or paid massage (bonus massage some essential oils like lavender on)
- Herbal topical relief cream (like arnica-based or Deep Heat)
- Gentle walk (seems counterproductive but often helps my neck and back, the key word is gentle)
- A swim
- Distraction (funny videos, phone a pick me up friend)

- Stretching (seriously, do this several times a day!).

If you're interested in a printable version of this list with a template for creating your a pain management plan, see my Etsy Store – MelissavFibromyalgia.

57

What I do:
Pacing and Boundaries

Pacing is a word often thrown about, yet it is difficult to implement. Especially if you are trying to live adjacent to normal. Even more so if the people in your life don't understand the consequences if you don't manage your energy well.

The pain-fatigue cycle is a vicious one – you can be exhausted due to high pain levels, and high pain levels lead to exhaustion.

Mounds of literature (and sources) on Fibromyalgia include pacing (see the website *The Pain Toolkit*), a core non-medicinal treatment. A part of what you can do in cognitive behavioural therapy (another prominent Fibromyalgia treatment) is to keep a diary of your activities for the purposes of finding limits and trying to stick to them.

A lot of my learning in this journey has smacked me upside the head, often after I've forgotten a lesson for a while. One of the first things I realised when I first cut down my work hours was that there are multiple benefits for me to finishing work at 3pm. While I'm unable to keep my brain and body sitting at the computer at this point, they do respond well to a brief rest and then a change in activity.

A fellow Fibromyalgia fighter, Anne Leppert, shared her tools for using pacing strategies to manage her symptoms in her article *Controlling Symptoms Through Pacing* on the CFIDS Self Help website. Things such as listening to your body, keeping a log of activities, focusing on sustainability and more - and I ought to be emulating these.

The concept of balancing activity and rest became integral to surviving when I was pregnant. I just couldn't physically sustain the crash and burn style I'm used to.

Meditation has supercharged my biggest rest period in a day – about 20-30 minutes is perfect. For the rest, I'll just sit quietly, with a book if I can.

It is difficult to ascertain your limits as they change day to day and season to season. But you can pay attention and begin to keep a note of your activity levels and pain levels and patterns will emerge.

Boundaries become important once you have recognised your limits and your pacing requirements. Sometimes, you'll need to fight for them.

Here are some tips to help:

- Keep to your desired bedtime, no matter what others may say.
- Take a 10 minute Yoga Nidra or body scan meditation in the car after work and before picking the child (or children) up if you are not at home during the day to snatch a rest.
- Find a stretch that you always find particularly delicious and do it a few times a day.
- Utilise pacing tools when doing computer work (and good ergonomics always!)
- Create an exercise plan and slowly work up, allowing for extra tired/painful days.
- Learn that you need to look after yourself. Put that oxygen mask on yourself before you help others with theirs!
- Grab any opportunity to do a meditation/hobby/exercise you love.
- Try to listen to your poor body when it screams "no!" But always expect slightly more.

Finding and respecting our energy envelope is crucial to surviving when we have 70, 60, 50 or less percentage of the energy levels that most of the people around us do. For me, this was and still continues to be an important part of my wellness plan.

Central Sensitivity/ Overactive Nervous System

A lot of research suggests that Fibromyalgia is the result of central nervous system dysfunction – specifically an overactive nervous system, stressing and exhausting the brain (Dennis W. Dobritt, *Fibromyalgia – A Brief Overview*)[10]. Other literature suggests that the chronic pain causes the central nervous system to go into overdrive. However you look at it, the nervous system appears to be involved.

The theory of autonomic nervous system dysfunction resonates with me as a big part of the puzzle – but not the entire answer.

A lot of programmes are popping up and claiming to "cure" chronic pain (Lightning Process, Curable app, the CFS Unraveled programme, various books with similar programmes) based upon the idea of retraining the brain. If these programmes are the entire answer for someone, I am happy

---

[10] Dennis W. Dobritt, DO, DABPM, FIPP. *Fibromyalgia - A Brief Overview (a presentation).* Retrieved from www.michigan.gov/documents/mdch/fibroacpsm_246421_7.pdf

for them. But mostly they are going to be one part of the puzzle.

Recently, I read Dr David Hanscom's book *Back in Control*, which outlines his programme for recovery from chronic pain[11]. It is heavily based upon rewiring the brain, but he also includes several other key components – including sleep. He emphasizes how important sleep is and believes that before a person can be successful with treating chronic pain, they must be sleeping well. I don't agree with all of his message, but I do like the fact that he recognizes the multiple components that are part of chronic pain-based illnesses. It is worth a read.

There are theories of anxiety and depression causing, or being the result of, Fibromyalgia as well. As usual, nothing is universal. Throwing people with Fibromyalgia on antidepressants (even without a diagnosis of depression) has long been the staple of some medical professionals; it certainly happens a lot here in New Zealand. But that really doesn't improve their quality of life or their condition. Depression and anxiety are just other parts of the puzzle for a lot of us.

---

[11] Dr David Hansom, MD. 2016. Back in Control. Vertus Press.

One of the key things I learnt from the first pain specialist I saw was about central sensitization. He helped me to see that by not treating my pain appropriately (I had a thing about avoiding medicines and try to take as little as possible), I was causing more pain – I was changing physiologically as a response to the ongoing pain and causing my nervous system to go into overdrive. So in addition to treating my pain, I needed to calm my nervous system down.

Luckily for me, prior to learning about this theory, I had already laid the ground work and made great progress with my overactive nervous system. Through meditation, which I have been practicing for a few years now, I no longer react as strongly to things that would have made my heart pound, breathing quicken and have me looking for the exit. Things that used to make me anxious no longer do. I also have the tools to calm myself down when my nervous system does go into overdrive. If I notice that I am getting wound up and my heartrate is climbing rapidly, I will quietly take several deep, gentle breaths, immediately calming my system. When I am feeling overwhelmed overall, I will sneak away to my room and meditate.

Meditation and mindfulness are great ways to help train your brain to calm down. Dr Hanscom also recommends free writing once or twice a day for five or ten minutes and then ripping up the page as a way of creating separation from issues. Some might also benefit from counselling or specific work on trauma-induced anxiety.

What I do: Meditation

I am acutely interested in the benefits of meditation for those with chronic illnesses. Yoga Nidra, a guided meditation, makes a real difference to my day. After a 20-minute session, my pain levels can drop to as low as 4/10 and decrease my fatigue levels to a similar place. The effects help me get through the busy evening period with my kids.

It's not easy to carve out 20 uninterrupted minutes. However, when I see a gap, I snatch it up.

As I mentioned earlier, a theory about Fibromyalgia is that the sympathetic nervous system (fight-or-flight response) may be stuck in overdrive[12]. Meditation promotes a calming of this system, allowing the parasympathetic nervous system to activate.

Some of the benefits of meditation are probably due to 20 minutes of lying down; using my heat pack on my neck; a break from noise; time alone; complete focus on my body, accepting it as it is (mindfulness); not struggling to nap,

---

[12] Martinez-Martinez et al. (2014). *Sympathetic nervous system dysfunction in fibromyalgia, chronic fatigue syndrome, irritable bowel syndrome, and interstitial cystitis: a review of case-control studies.* PubMed. Retrieved from www.ncbi.nlm.nih.gov/pubmed

which I can't, so using the time calmly and effectively; and the body's response to complete relaxation, allowing the sympathetic nervous system to slow down.

Meditation is an important tool for well-being that I keep close; it is something that transcends simple pain/fatigue relief and gives me time to focus on myself as a whole. My san culpa (mantra/goal of practice) is "*I am healing; I am well.*" In her book *Superhealing: Engaging Your Mind, Body, and Spirit to Create Optimal Health and Well-Being* (2013), Dr Elaine R. Ferguson, MD, agrees with this:

> *"Practicing this [mindfulness] meditation affects your mind, brain, body and behavior in ways that promote whole-person health."*

It's vital that we don't neglect our spiritual and emotional components of self in the quest for relief from physical issues. I feel there's a close tie between my emotions and my pain/fatigue levels. Fear or sadness have an effect on my sympathetic nervous system, which affects the body physically. So I am researching both body and mind effects on Fibromyalgia.

Meditation and Me

It took me a while to appreciate meditation – years, in fact, for me to consider giving up precious reading time for it.

Suddenly, in 2014, I read a book about mindfulness meditation and found a YouTube video of a Yoga Nidra session – it's called *Yoga Nidra – Deeply Restorative Guided Relaxation/Meditation* – that I particularly liked (avoiding the spiritual/religious aspects of it) and then I was away running.

I have meditations, body scans and Yoga Nidra of varying lengths that I switch between as I like. I also use the body scan technique most nights to relax into sleep. The focus on the breath is like second nature to fall into. Now, when I am stuck awake in the middle of the night (usually after the kids have woken me) instead of tossing and turning in frustration, I do a body scan meditation. Not stressing about not sleeping combined with the effects of the deep rest are both restorative and usually lead back to sleep.

When I was pregnant and desperately tired and sore, meditation made a huge difference to my quality of life. Sometimes, I would even catch 5-10 minutes of sleep after the meditation finished and feel uniquely restored. On days when I have not slept well, it is deeply soothing to be able to rest completely without wishing I could nap.

The benefits of meditation have pervaded all facets of my life – I no longer get anxious without due cause. I feel profoundly calmed by the fact that I can attain deep rest in the face of constant fatigue and chronic insomnia, and I adore that this coping mechanism is freely available to me any time, any place.

Meditation Options

You can:

- Simply focus on your breath for a few moments. How you breathe in, how the breath feels a little warmer on the way out. How your body feels when you exhale. How your breaths get a little longer as you relax. Don't push anything, just observe.
- Do your own body scan meditation – by quietly thinking of each part of your body in turn, noticing the feeling in each, accepting it, willing that part to relax and moving to the next.
- Do progressive relaxation – by tensing and releasing each part of your body in turn, you can encourage it

to relax deeply. As an example, you could start with your feet, tense and release, your lower legs, upper legs, glutes, abdomen, arms, face.

- Guided meditations – YouTube has a heap available including Yoga Nidra, mindfulness meditations, meditation specific to pain or fatigue etc.

Recommended Reads

- *You Are Not Your Pain: Using Mindfulness to Relieve Pain, Reduce Stress and Restore Wellbeing – an Eight Week Program* by Vidyamala Birch and Danny Penman (2013)
- *Back in Control: A Surgeon's Roadmap out of Chronic Pain* by David Hanscom

What I do:
Yoga for Fibromyalgia

Type "Yoga for Fibromyalgia" into Google and you will find a wealth of information trails to follow. Countless blogs and articles cover the benefits of yoga, meditation, and mindfulness for people with Fibromyalgia.

The crossover of yoga into the Western world has resulted in a more mainstream practice and scientific research backing up what practitioners have known for years. There's even research that has found encouraging correlations between regular yoga practice and decreases in pain, fatigue, and sleep problems (see the article *School of Medicine Research Indicates Yoga Can Counteract Fibromyalgia* on the OHSU website). The styles of yoga recommended for those with Fibromyalgia are relatively relaxing. Restorative yoga is highly recommended.

A sequence I created with a yoga instructor has given me the basis for regular practice, with modifications for days where I haven't the energy or pain levels to cope with a full sequence, and for days when I feel I can push a little further.

I have some gentle, restorative poses that I enact naturally, especially legs on a chair (see Mia Park's article *Restorative Yoga Pose: Legs on a Chair* on Yoga International) and child's pose (see the video *Child's Pose* on Health.com).

After more than a decade of learning to live well with Fibromyalgia, perhaps the most valuable learning I possess is the ability to tune in to my body. I am constantly analysing what works, what doesn't, what's causing what pain, and what helps which body parts. I have brought this into my yoga journey, which has had ebbs and flows over the amount of time I've dealt with the pain.

The value of yoga for a body with pain and fatigue can be found in:

- The awareness of what you are doing with your body in each pose, consciously engaging the correct muscles, taking the correct stretch or benefit on offer
- The basis of the breath. Breathing is key to yoga and to accessing the parasympathetic nervous system[13]. Even the stretches encourage full use of the breath, offering relaxation benefits to stretches

---

[13] Joe Miller. (n.d.). *The Benefits of Yoga on the Parasympathetic Nervous System*. The Nest. Retrieved from the website http://woman.thenest.com.

- The invitation to be outside of usual mind chatter – it's so easy to be lost in the movement, the breath, and the experience of the pose
- The gentle strengthening – a favoured pose, Downward Facing Dog, utilises all the key muscle groups.
- The ease of fitting practice in. Somedays, it can be 20 minutes on the mat, engaged in a flowing sequence. Others, it can be a few key stretches in snippets of minutes. On yet others, it can be one restorative pose for 10 minutes. Corpse pose can be used when sleep is being elusive, with or without a body scan relaxation.

The practice of yoga also includes many options and I definitely make use of the tools it offers. And some of these yoga tools include:

- Sequences focused on strengthening – I do a modified sun salutation sequence with additions when I feel I can. Clint Paddison recommends for those with Rheumatoid Arthritis[14].

---

[14] Clint Paddison. (2015). *7 Restorative Yoga Poses for Balance of Body, Mind, Spirit.* Rheumatoid Arthritis. Retrieved from the website https://www.paddisonprogram.com.

- Stretching poses – *Child's Pose* (video) on Health.com.
- Restorative sequences or one-off poses (see Kelly McGonigal's article *Restorative Yoga for Chronic Pain* on the Yoga International website).
- Yoga Nidra, guided meditation "yogic sleep" (see Elaine Gavalas's article *3 Yoga Nidra Health Benefits* on Huffpost).
- Yogic breathing (see *Mastering the Yogic Breath* by Daniel Scott).

Yoga Nidra is especially healing for me. I come back to again and again. My ideal yoga practice would look like this: sun salutations first thing, gentle yogic stretches at work, Yoga Nidra after work, and legs on the chair pose in the evening. Or any one of these in a day. I never do all of them.

Perhaps one of the best parts of yoga for Fibromyalgia is that you can fine tune it to your experience, your day, your mood. If the fatigue is bad and post exertional malaise has been plaguing you, you can choose a few poses and take breaks. If a particular body part has been upset, you can gently stretch all the muscles around it to free it up. If you're desperate for a break from your mind and its constant noise, you can do a guided Yoga Nidra session and let the voice take over for a time.

Resource List

- Yoga for Chronic Pain: 7 Steps to Aid Recovery from Fibromyalgia with Yoga is a book by Kayla Kuran – She is a yoga therapist who has Fibromyalgia.

- Yoga Nidra meditation for healing (a YouTube video) – this is one of my regular practices (I do Yoga Nidra daily).

- Sleep Santosha YouTube channel has so many great videos for spoonies.

What I do:
Gentle Exercise

The number one rule of fighting Fibromyalgia is to keep moving, even when it seems near impossible. If stretching is all you can manage, do it. If you can walk down your hallway and back, do it. If you can do a series of Yoga Sun Salutations, do it.

Movement keeps the muscles moving and strong. It's much harder to bring the muscles back from atrophy than it is to keep using them.

Of course, I don't mean you should be launching into graded exercise therapy and pushing your way up to functional improvements to the detriment of your quality of life. Quality of life is what all of this is about.

Research

A meta-analysis of the impact of aerobic exercise on Fibromyalgia symptoms revealed positive impacts on pain, fatigue and mood. However, the effects were lost post treatment –

exercise must be done regularly (see Winfried Häuser et al's article *Efficacy of Different Types of Aerobic Exercise in Fibromyalgia Syndrome*).

It is recommended that we begin below our ability level and then build up slowly. The goal of exercise is to improve our quality of life. Therefore, increasing your exercise capacity but leaving pain levels similar or increased, is not considered success. The quote below from the article *Exercise Therapy for Fibromyalgia* (2011) explains the best method:

"The intensity and duration of exercise sessions should be reduced when significant post-exertion pain or fatigue is experienced and the intensity increased by 10% after 2 weeks of exercise without exacerbating symptoms."

Moderate intensity exercise is usually recommended. Warm water exercise is particularly helpful due to the water providing a weightlessness. Walking, strength training and yoga are all regularly recommended types of exercise.

What I Do

Walking is a means of exercise that has yet to fail me. There are multiple benefits to going for a walk in fresh air and warm sunshine. However, if going around the block is too much of a challenge, then walk down the hallway and back, to the letterbox and back – start where you are. Each time I've been knocked back health-wise, I have started where I could and built up from there. If walking is out of reach, stretch. Using your muscles is important.

When I was heavily pregnant with my first son, I listened to all the information that said keeping active would help with labour and forgot the advice to rest while I could. It was silly, I don't even know how I got around the block, but I pushed myself to do it right until the last day I was pregnant.

In the third trimester with my second son, I couldn't do more than a gentle walk pushing a pushchair around the shops. A pelvis issue made it impossible. But once I healed enough from that, several months after he was born, I was back at walking. First to the end of the street and back, then a little further until I was back at my 20-30 minute walks.

Prior to my boys, I preferred Pilates as my resistance-based exercise. Since then, I have switched to yoga. I really enjoy the breath based work; it's simultaneously calming and energising. There's more information about yoga and its benefit for Fibromyalgia in the *What I do: Yoga* chapter.

A few years ago, when Noah was small, my knee randomly became severely painful. I remember being in agony trying to walk from the lounge to the kitchen. The physiotherapist said it was due to the smallest muscle of my quadriceps that had been underutilised while pregnant and having a tiny baby – presumably due to the lack of Pilates or yoga. Like a good girl, I did the stretches prescribed to the letter. I was still in severe pain. So I took Noah down to the nearest swimming pool and walked across the pool and back holding him. The weight of the water sured up my leg enabling pain free movement. Then we soaked in the family spa (a spa heated to a lower temperature so it was suitable for children). It was bliss.

Here's some of my key advice:

- Move somehow
- Don't overdo it
- Choose something you enjoy
- Hot water is divine

What I do: Physiotherapy and Acupuncture

You can learn to do a lot for yourself, but a good treatment with a compassionate, knowledgeable practitioner is truly a blessing. My physiotherapist is the only person I tell most of my daily symptoms to. It's a gift to speak it out loud and have someone understand.

Research appears to be mixed about the benefits of acupuncture on Fibromyalgia symptoms. An analysis undertaken in 2013 (*Acupuncture for Treating Fibromyalgia* on PubMed) looked at nine trials with 395 participants and found this:

"Acupuncture is probably better than non-acupuncture treatment in reducing pain and stiffness and improving overall well-being and fatigue; acupuncture without electrical stimulation probably does not reduce pain or improve fatigue, overall well-being or sleep."

Traditional acupuncture didn't help me either, but the use of acupuncture needles in trigger points does. In the case of trigger points, a lot of support appears for treatment by a physical therapist. In the article *Information About Trigger Points and Their Treatment* (n.d.), it states:

> *"Doctors may use local anaesthetic, saline, or cortisone injections, but acupuncture needling, use of a cold spray whilst stretching the muscle, or specific trigger point massage also works. Some physiotherapists or masseurs have a real knack in treating TPs [trigger point]."*

Recently, I learnt (after over a decade) that my neck pain is caused by MPS: severe, recurring trigger points. So acupuncture needles in the trigger points in my neck and shoulders really help me. To the point that I cannot go too long without treatment and nothing else will hold off the increasing pain and tension, resulting in dizziness, nausea and severe headaches.

Find a physical therapy that offers you (with your unique experience) relief. Some key physical therapy are physiotherapy, massage, osteopathy, chiropractic, and reflexology

Through a lot of experience, research, trial and error, I know that I need neck tractions (stretches) before and after acupuncture needles placed into the trigger points on my sub occipital and upper trapezius points.

I use self-trigger point therapy (I jab my thumb or finger into the trigger point for as long as I can hold it for up to a couple of minutes), stretch regularly and use my trigger point massage cane to get those spots that are hard to reach myself and to get more deeply into those key points. I also do all of the things I write about in this book: ply my neck with heat in the form of hot showers, heat pack and non-medicated hot rubs.

Still, I need to see the physiotherapist for this treatment within three weeks or I begin to struggle with sleep. The pain and tightness will keep me awake, drive me to change pillows multiple times, get my heat pack, and, if necessary, take medicine.

I always start the day stiff, but when my neck is worse, it can be so stiff and tight that I can hardly move it, and the accompanying headache is relentless. If I let it escalate too far, then I'll end up miserable and unable to function. At this level, only muscle relaxants can work.

I am thankful I have worked this out, which enables me to limit the pain relief medications I need to take as well as improving my quality of life. Try to take some time to find what may provide you with relief. Some people swear by regular massages, others by osteopathy. I have found that a lot of these therapies overlap – my physiotherapist can do some chiropractic adjustments if needed and an osteopath will utilise massage, craniosacral therapy, and adjustments, too.

What I Do: Medicine – Low Dose Naltrexone

Medicines are a tricky business when it comes to Fibromyalgia. What works for one may not work for another. In addition, side effects are generally pretty noticeable and often the effects of the drug wear off after time.

LDN has been such an amazing find for me. Being able to achieve better sleep and all of the positive offshoots of that is something I am grateful for every single day.

About LDN

LDN works in the endocannabinoid system. It temporarily blocks the receptors encouraging the body to make more endorphins. There is research suggesting that a cause of Fibromyalgia could be due to an endocannabinoid deficiency.[15] Given how well it helps me, it could be a plausible explanation.

---

[15] Ethan B. Russo. 2016. *Clinical Endocannabinoid Deficiency Reconsidered: Current Research Supports the Theory in Migraine, Fibromyalgia, Irritable Bowel, and Other Treatment-Resistant* Syndromes. 1(1): 154–165. doi: 10.1089/can.2016.0009.

However Fibromyalgia may originate, I like the fact that LDN essentially spurs your own body into action and that there are few side effects. There is also plenty of research and patient evidence. I believe that patient-evidence (this term, which I love, was coined by Julia Schopick in her book Honest Medicine) is very important. That's your voice, not the researcher's voice.

An interesting thing about LDN is that different doses help different people and it can take widely varied amounts of time to work. So these research studies currently taking place (as below) that use a standard dose of 4.5mg for about eight weeks are not going to give us the full picture. They are a great start, however.

Research by Dr Jarred Younger has been promising. Younger, along with Luke Parkitny and David McLain, started with a tiny study and found positive results; approximately 65% of patients have experienced clinically significant results[16]. In 2017, Dr Jarred Younger was involved with

---

[16] Jarred Younger, Luke Parkitny, & David McLain, *The Use of Low-Dose Naltrexone (LDN) as a Novel Anti-Inflammatory Treatment for Chronic Pain* (2014), retrieved from ncbi.nlm.nih.gov/pmc

a bigger study, and early results sound promising – I look forward to the final results[17].

As a member of an active group called *What Works for Fibromyalgia* and two groups about low dose naltrexone on Facebook, I have seen many testimonies from people with Fibromyalgia experiencing changes due to LDN ranging from mildly beneficial to miraculous. There are also those for whom it does not work or they do not try it for long enough – this is not a quick fix for most.

Further information on how LDN works is well-explained by Dr Jill Carnahan, MD, in her article *Low Dose Naltrexone: The New Treatment You've Never Heard Of* on her website, which includes many links to research.

Low dose naltrexone came on my radar in 2016, and after consuming all of the research and anecdotal evidence about its impact on Fibromyalgia, I earmarked it for my major experiment post-baby (I had baby December 2016 and nursed until April 2017 – when I began).

---

[17] UAB, College of Arts and Science. (n.d.) Current Projects. Retrieved from https://cas.uab.edu/

LDN and Pregnancy –
An Area to Research Carefully

I learned afterward that it is *potentially* safe to take LDN until the 37th week. I believe this is to be because you generally go into labour anytime from 37-42 weeks and you may need opioids during the labour – I did for all of my labours.

There are fertility clinics that use LDN specifically to help women with autoimmune conditions to maintain a pregnancy. So there are a lot of women who have been given it for pregnancy. But this is a decision you and your doctor must make after looking at the available evidence, which includes anecdotal evidence as research into medicines during pregnancy would be unethical.

There are no long term studies as of yet. As with all medicine use in pregnancy, it would be a matter of balancing cost versus benefits. Would the LDN help more than the potential risks? I did this in conjunction with my doctor and a specialist for amitriptyline for all of my pregnancies – and we came to the conclusion that I was already sleeping so poorly due to pregnancy that coming off it would only add to the stress on my body.

Dr Phil Boyle presents his findings in a presentation – *Low Dose Naltrexone in Pregnancy* (n.d.) – showing the comparison of outcomes between those in his clinic that used LDN and those that didn't, and the results were fairly positive. On the flipside of that, a study on animals using LDN during pregnancy was not-so positive, as documented on the LDN Now website.

It is considered potentially safe for breastfeeding – this is discussed on Drugs.com discusses this in the article *Naltrexone Use While Breasting* (n.d.):

> *"Limited data indicate that naltrexone is minimally excreted into breast milk. If naltrexone is required by the mother, it is not a reason to discontinue breastfeeding."*

Please note: This is a finding on the usual dose of Naltrexone, often used to help detox off drugs.

LDN and Me

I believed if I could experience a 30% (this is considered clinically significant and therefore as success) decrease in pain and fatigue, my life would change. I could be a mama, a wife, do my work and have some form of a life outside that and not pay with such significant levels of pain, fatigue and other side effects of the Fibromyalgia.

I can only share research and what works or doesn't work for me. We are all unique and react differently. If you're interested in LDN, then please read the research and information and then discuss it with your doctor.

I began LDN in April 2017. I had a small baby who had reflux and didn't sleep well. It was a trial by fire for LDN. I began on 0.5mg and titrated up slowly, as I could manage. Side effects included vivid dreams for the first few nights at a new dose. I also experienced a surge of ulcers and cold sores early on. I believe this was my immune system coming back online appropriately.

The effects were subtle. After a few months, I accidentally skipped two nights close to each other and found myself feeling like I were hit by a truck carrying a whopping amount of fatigue.

After several months, I noted an increase in stamina, slightly decreased fatigue and slightly decreased neck pain. It was a challenge to note because the second I have more energy, I use it. I am my own worst enemy at times. My average pain levels went from around 4-7/10 down to 3-5/10 with higher being a flare up caused by ignoring my limits.

Without external interference (in the guise of, say, a cute squishy baby), the combination of amitriptyline and LDN appeared to help me sleep slightly better – I often attained blocks of sleep in a row, sometimes up to five or six hours. This almost never happened previously.

As I wrote in the conclusion of my one year experiment on my blog there are five main ways that LDN helps me:

Sleep

First and foremost is sleep. For the ten years or so prior to LDN, I had not slept in more than one hour blocks, that's rarely completing a whole sleep cycle, therefore my body was in chronic deep sleep deprivation. Since LDN, I can sleep in two, three, four or even five hour blocks! I am so grateful for this, I can't even tell you. I believe this is what has created the other benefits.

Please do note that I still enact my sleep hygiene list daily.

Pain

Since about nine months into treatment, I have noticed a reduction in neck pain. Neck pain has been a 24/7 issue for over 10 years. In 2017, while starting LDN, I learnt that my neck issue is actually MPSsrome. After throwing the severe, recurring "muscle knots" (trigger points) into the fibro basket, I finally had an answer. The physiotherapist has been helping me to work on these trigger points through intramuscular needling (gently inserting a tiny needle into the trigger point and letting it relax a little) and neck mobilisations. This, and the sleep (potentially reducing the Fibromyalgia), has helped. My pain levels were 6-8/10 with severe headaches (with dizziness and nausea) daily back in 2010 before I started this journey. Just prior to LDN they were approximately 4-6/10 with occasional severe headaches. In early 2018, after one year on LDN, the average was 3-4/10 with the occasional spike to 5/6 with a bad headache and was usually when I'd overdone it.

Emotional

If you haven't lived with pain that interrupts sleep, interferes with daily life all day, every day for over a decade or been unable to sleep for more than an hour at a time for about the same length of time – it'll be hard to convey the depth of impact on my emotional well-being.

Not fighting to sleep at 3am, not swapping pillows, getting my heat pack, applying pain cream and basically not sleeping due to unrelenting pain is huge for me.

My quality of life is so much better. I never let myself lose hope, but it was dwindling. This was a necessary win.

Stamina

Slowly my stamina increased. Activities that used to wipe me out can be tolerated for longer. I can exercise slightly more. I can do slightly more.

Having had a baby with reflux, I feel I coped exceptionally well and that is down to LDN.

Fatigue

Fatigue is the second of my two worst symptoms (neck pain being the first). Yes, that's "is" not "was". It's improved but I still have a limited energy envelope. I can get through the day on a 15 minute meditation and a brief sit down with the heat pack. I still can't physically stay up past 10pm or out past 7pm and that's a fair trade off to me.

Another interesting effect was that I lost five kilograms. I was at my pre-Fibromyalgia weight (although not my previous body fat percentage) prior to my third pregnancy.

LDN and My Third Pregnancy

In February 2018 I found out that I was pregnant with my third baby. I immediately went back over the research around pregnancy and LDN, took it to my doctor and was prepared to plead my case. Getting some sleep and having less pain was surely a good recipe for pregnancy. Thankfully my doctor agreed and I stayed on my 4mg dose.

Aside from slightly increased nausea in the first trimester than the first two times, the experience was worlds apart.

At week 11 I noted that at the same point in my second pregnancy I was already miserable, struggling to sleep and taking codeine to try and get some rest. This time I was working 24 hours a week and looking after two tiny children – one of whom still woke frequently at night.

At week 20, despite symphysis pubis disorder being a real bother, read: my pelvis separated too far, my hips were asymmetrical, my hospital physiotherapist wanted me on crutches and I was in consistent back and pelvis pain with limited mobility – the Fibromyalgia was being relatively kind to me.

My neck and shoulders were starting to feel the impact of side sleeping, but I was still sleeping in two or three hour blocks. I was thankful for this every single day.

I tracked my experience so that I could share it with others who needed it as there is so little research available in this area. There is no registry that I could find that tracks LDN use in pregnancy and there are no experiments on pregnant women using medicine for ethical reasons. In my LDN Facebook groups, I did speak to many women who stayed on for their entire pregnancies, went back on for nursing and had healthy babies and pleasant experiences.

One issue to consider was when to go off in case of the need for opioids during labour. Generally, a woman can deliver between 37 and 42 weeks, but I didn't want to be off LDN for that long. I had to balance the fact that previously I had had long early labours requiring pethidine and that I might need pain relief after the delivery for the symphysis pubis disorder (I was in exceedingly high levels of pain last time). I tentatively decided to go off at 37 weeks.

At 37 weeks and 3 days, I stopped dosing. By the second night, sleep was more difficult to attain; getting back to sleep after being woken by the four-year-old, then the husband was hard. So, on top of a lingering cold, low iron levels, and being heavily pregnant, I was exhausted.

Thankfully, baby came at 38 weeks and 3 days. I did need an epidural with some narcotics in. I restarted LDN five days postpartum. I feel like I dealt very well with the sleep deprivation and physical strain of the early months. Though, by 10 weeks, I was starting to struggle and needed to be actively managing the neck and shoulders again. During week 10, I suffered my first severe headache with nausea in months and took my first dose of ibuprofen since the after pains subsided within the first two weeks. When the baby let me sleep, I fell asleep easily and slept deeply which made all the difference.

What I do:
Medicine – Amitriptyline

As I mentioned, prior to LDN, amitriptyline was the only thing to help me sleep.

The mechanism of amitriptyline is to increase the level of serotonin, hypothesized to be low in people with Fibromyalgia.

In *Fibromyalgia and Muscle Pain: Your Guide to Self-Treatment* (2015) by Leon Chaitow ND, DO, the section on medication is very small, but he does mention amitriptyline as one of the most useful medicines prescribed for Fibromyalgia.

"Studies involving various forms of antidepressant medication tend to support the use of amitriptyline (25 to 50 mg daily), with pain scores, stiffness, sleep and fatigue symptoms all improving on average, but by no means in all sufferers."

I was put on amitriptyline before I was diagnosed by a locum GP I saw only once. Without knowing what it does or why I was put on it, it turned out to be the best foundation for my journey to wellness. I started on 50mg per night and stayed on this dose until I questioned its efficacy – I slept poorly – and my Fitbit sleep chart was always alight with the colours of restlessness or awake time. I barely cobbled together an hour at a time.

One December, I decided to experiment with going off it. I slowly reduced my dose – this is not a medicine that you can just stop. I went much more slowly than my doctor suggested, and this served me well. On the way down, I noted that at 30 and 25mg, I experienced the same level of benefit with getting to sleep as at 50mg. When I got lower than that, I began to sleep extremely poorly, to feel a lot more pain, and to get constant headaches. I endured two weeks completely off it, including trialling 5HTP (a supplement said to help with sleep), and I was miserable.

Declaring amitriptyline as useful, I went back to 25mg. It was a good thing to have tested its worth after nearly a decade on it because there are side effects and risks. However, learning I could halve the dose was a good lesson.

In 2018, after the birth of my third baby, I decided to stop taking it as I was confident the LDN was helping enough and I was going to experience sleep deprivation anyway (from the newborn baby). I quietly stopped taking it, unsure if it would stick. After a week, I acknowledged to myself that I was ok. I then announced it to my husband – I was so excited to finally be off a medicine I didn't feel I needed anymore after more than a decade on it.

I am thankful it helped me when nothing else did but with the LDN the cost vs benefit analysis no longer worked for me.

What I do: Supplements

Supplements are a tricky area to write about. Requirements are very individual. There are several supplements that are broadly recommended for Fibromyalgia patients. However, a lot of them are a waste of money, unless your body needs them.

Dr Teitelbaum, Dr Liptan, Dr Brady, and numerous other doctors writing books and articles about Fibromyalgia recommend liberal use of supplements and natural remedies. Anecdotally, patients will swear by certain ones.

Unless you have a good functional medicine doctor or naturopath who can do reliable testing and tell you exactly what your body needs, you're flying blind.

As a person who has tried a lot of supplements based upon research, doctors' recommendations and a (disappointing) naturopath (who encouraged me to spend hundreds of dollars to be "cured"), I can tell you what I do take.

There are countless articles to wade through. Here, I outline some articles recommending supplements for Fibromyalgia.

Some of the most commonly mentioned supplements are:

- Acetyl L-carnitine
- Magnesium
- Fish oil
- Turmeric and black pepper
- Vitamin D3
- 5-HTP
- SAMe
- CoQ10 (energy)
- D-Ribose (energy)

In his article *8 Natural Ways to Overcome Fibromyalgia Symptoms* (n.d.), Dr Axe lists the main symptoms of Fibromyalgia, treatment options, foods to eat to gain good nutrients, such as melatonin, and natural treatments.

Karen Lee Richards discusses the diminished energy present for those with Fibromyalgia and lists several options in her article *8 Energy-Boosting Supplements for Fight Fibromyalgia Fatigue* (2011) on the Fibromyalgia Treatment Group website.

On that same website, there's an article called *10 Herbs and Supplements to Try for Fibromyalgia Pain* (n.d.), and it focuses on pain and adds Alpha Lipoic Acid, Rhodiola Rosea and Butterbur in addition to the above list.

Fibro Daze's article *14 Supplements That May Help Fibromyalgia* (2014) diverges a little from the other articles and adds malic acid, B complex, NADH, DHEA, probiotics and melatonin. The author, Sue, who has Fibromyalgia, takes these, alongside a multivitamin and milk thistle.

Dr Teitelbaum's website *EndFatigue* has a Nutrition Guide with a list of herbals, vitamins, minerals and other supplements with links to further information about them and recommended dosage.

I have read Dr Teitelbaum's books and a lot of the articles on his website and it all makes sense to me. I feel I would have made more progress if doctors would help me tackle the sleep issue – he believes (if necessary) a couple of low dose medicines to aid sleep for several months is very efficacious to healing[18]. I like his book *The Fatigue and Fibromyalgia Solution* (2013).

The few supplements I currently take include:

- Magnesium Oil – for potential deficiency and potential help with sleep.
- A good powdered multivitamin
- Probiotics

I also like:

---

[18] Dr. Jacob Teitelbaum. (2013). *The Fatigue and Fibromyalgia Solution.* Avery.

- Moringa Powder – for nutritional support, it has 18 amino acids, is a good source of vitamins and minerals.

- MSM

It is a good idea when trying new supplements to add one thing at a time and to track the outcomes. Please keep in mind, it does take time for these to build up in the system. I found with MSM (a supplement I was taking prior to LDN kicking in) it took about six weeks to notice a difference.

Supplement Log	
Supplements	
Dates Trialled	
Dosage(s)	
Effects	
Outcome	

What I do: Brain Fog

There's a pernicious symptom of living with Fibromyalgia that can fall into the background of the twin peaks of pain and fatigue. Something that affects our everyday lives and we may not even realise it is a thing.

Brain fog or cognitive dysfunction (a very unattractive term, but there it is) – it can strike during any conversation, any task, any time.

I can't do confrontations because the stress causes me to forget how to stand up for myself. All the words or well-articulated statements I'd have written down become buried in fog when I try to access them in the moment. Even subjects I'm well researched on become minefields when reaching through my memory for the information. Which is part of why I write everything down.

There's been a thousand conversations where I'm reaching for simple words that blew away a moment before I want them. There have been even more times when I say one thing when I mean another. Sometimes I know I've done it, but often I don't. Occasionally, I'll realise later. As someone who loves words and writing, it's more than a little upsetting.

Brain fog was thought to be another thing that is all in our heads, but "a 2015 study in *Arthritis Care and Research* found that fibro fog is a real issue. In a study of 60 individuals – 30 with fibromyalgia and 30 without fibromyalgia – researchers found various impairments of attention and memory in fibromyalgia patients when compared with healthy controls. What remains unclear is what is causing the cognitive challenges" (*Fibro Fog: Sleep, Brain Dysfunction Likely Culprits for Cognitive Difficulties Associated with Fibromyalgia*, the Arthritis Foundation website). It is thought as many as 50% of Fibromyalgia patients struggle with it, perhaps more.

Brain fog has been theorized to be caused by poor sleep, the nervous system being off-kilter, stress and anxiety, and pain severity. Though, they really don't know the cause yet.

Here's the way it can manifest:

- Climsiness/loss of spacial awareness
- Losing words
- Mixing up words
- Forgetting things
- Confusion (I've never experienced this but see how it could occur)

- Overwhelm (too many competing sensory inputs)
- Becoming easily distracted

Here's some things that help minimise brain fog:

- Get the best sleep you can get (something I have found and is supported by the literature – sleep really is king to managing Fibromyalgia symptoms)
- Pace activity and rest
- Manage pain
- Give yourself time and understanding

These are not small things for us to do. I spend a lot of time working on good sleep and managing pain, and brain fog is still a big factor in my life. However, it's far better to what it was when I was at my worst.

Here's some ways to combat brain fog's effects:

- Lists, write it all down – even before I was diagnosed or had any idea of why life was so much harder for me, I planned religiously and had lists upon lists.
- Routines, automatic pilot can be useful.

- Explain it to those around you often – I often tell my family that there is nothing more dear to me than a person who mercifully adds the right word in their own head for me or gives it to me gently.
- Check your medicines are not the culprits – sometimes, our medicines cause as many issues as they solve; it's good to be aware of what their side effects are so we can mitigate them.

Brain fog is just one of those things that come with chronic sleep deprivation, pain and fatigue, but there are many things we can do to compensate for it.

What I do: Passion

I am a willful person. Looking back at when I was struggling to work full-time, right before I made my major lifestyle changes, I wonder how I didn't pass out from the pain and fatigue each day. It was only my willfulness that kept me going. In order to fight constant pain and fatigue, one must have a reason to.

Once the brain fog that accompanies worse pain and the fatigue began to recede, I was able to begin to read again. It was a miracle of epic proportions to me that I had the energy again to read. Since then, I have read voraciously, about 80 books per year (as an estimate).

We might not be able to continue all of our previous hobbies; I certainly gave up the gym and dramatically reduced the amount of exercise I did in order to reduce a lot of my lower body pain.

But we must look to what we *can* do, not what we *can't*.

And despite limited energy levels that require us to do less than most, we still deserve to pursue a fulfilling hobby.

We need passion to keep us going through the fight, especially when the fight leaves us in bed in severe pain for a few days or weeks.

Take the time to remember what you love to do, think back to your childhood and something will come up. Think on what you would do if you suddenly had a whole day free. Make a list of things you love to do.

When I was just starting my recovery and reading was still a boon, I had a list of things I could do in ascending order of pain level. Something as simple as a hot cup of coffee while sitting on the deck in the early morning sun, or creating a page in a scrapbook, or talking to a dear friend on the phone. Make your list for when the lethargy hits, the pain level increases or the fatigue has you bed bound.

Don't let chronic illness take your goals. Reshape them, make new ones and plan for it.

My Favourite Authors

Jane Austen

Kate Morton

Belinda Alexandra

Cecelia Ahern

Sarah J Maas

Jennifer L Armentrout

Passion Template

What do I really enjoy to do?

What did I really enjoy as a child?

What would I do if fatigue/pain weren't a problem?

If I suddenly had a whole day free, what would I do?

What I do: Food

A lot of Fibromyalgia fighters swear by eating one way or the other. I have found that prioritising whole foods has been the only answer for me. I tried gluten free for eight weeks to no effect. I am currently mostly dairy free as it upsets my tummy.

I have looked into the vegetarian, the paleo, the anti-inflammatory, and the other diets recommended for Fibromyalgia and have noticed one main similarity: prioritising vegetables.

In her book *The Whole Health Life* (2016), Shannon Harvey writes about being well with a chronic illness that affects her gut. In her chapter on food, she outlines her research into the different diets and comes to a conclusion that I agree with:

"A diet rich in whole, plant-based foods is the way to go."

I believe it is worth doing a trial excluding certain foods, especially gluten, as I have heard enough stories of partial or full recovery for it to be worth an eight-week trial without it to be sure it is not a contributor for me.

The Mediterranean Diet is highly regarded – it prioritises fresh fruits and vegetables, whole grains, healthy fats, seafood and meats. You might like to research that further. For myself, my constant refrain is "food as fuel" – I need the energy for living, not for trying to process junky food. I focus on vegetables, fruits, whole grains, protein, etc., but I am not super strict. I have found no foods that make me feel noticeably better by avoiding them. With the exception of MSG, aspartame, etc., I don't eliminate foods unless they cause an intolerance/allergy for me or are of no nutritional value.

Several years ago, I realised that my body was trying to gain energy by driving me to consume carbohydrates – *a lot.* Ironically, the carbohydrates take lots of energy to process, thereby draining more energy and making me crave more food. By taking note of the food I was eating on a daily basis for a few weeks, I realised that I was consuming way too many carbohydrates, especially the white ones – with little to no nutritional value. The food diary showed me I was perpetuating a boom-bust cycle every few hours – eat carbohydrate, crash, consume again, crash again. When the fatigue increases, I do notice a craving for the white carbs, especially Chelsea buns – buns with cinnamon, raisins and a white or pink icing. It's been so obviously beneficial to me to avoid these, that it's usually not my first craving. But if it is, I easily make a swap for something better.

Sugar is another thing we consume too abundantly. Especially when we are tired. As opposed to trying to put myself on a strict diet to avoid sugar, I choose to focus on better food choices. By prioritising those foods mentioned above such as vegetables, fruits and whole grains – we leave less room for those processed, sugary, empty calorie, anti-nutrients we call food. As someone with a lot of coping mechanisms to enact every day, it is better to not make food a battleground.

My Favourite Beverages

Coffee

Chai tea latte

Peppermint tea

Chamomile tea

Peach iced tea

What I do: Support

This is a prickly topic for me.

This is something I've sorely missed out on and wish for you to have. When I was first diagnosed – and for a great many years after – the only person I spoke to who had even heard the term Fibromyalgia was my doctor. And she not only didn't help me at all, but she discouraged me from reducing my work hours as she believed I'd be disappointed that I'd still be sore and tired. Boy, was she wrong.

It's only recently that I've had a tiny team and most of them are virtual connections. If there is no one in real life, get a virtual crew – I like the solutions focused groups such as *What Works for Fibromyalgia* Facebook group – they provide a real sense of not doing it alone and all of them are fighting as hard as I am and have much to offer in advice.

I have had a profound longing to be witnessed, to not be alone. As I found when I had my babies, there was nothing worse than being completely alone, in pain, exhausted with a screaming baby. Even if the person can't help any of the issues, their presence, especially if it's my husband, soothes me.

My sister and younger brother, Luke, have both lent me a compassionate ear many times. For that I am grateful. Luke has also helped me a lot physically since I had my children. He will come and stay and help me through the evening rush hours when my husband works nightshift. He will do the dishes and vacuum. He has also spent hours and hours editing my writing and creating images for my blog and books. All Fibro People need a Lukie.

But nothing does fill the gap like someone who gets it. I highly recommend connecting with others who are fighting this journey. At the same time, I don't recommend people who are not actively fighting the Fibromyalgia and are maybe a little pessimistic – I would struggle letting someone vent and not being able to suggest anything to help. And listening to the same complaints over would be frustrating. Find what works for you and connect. Especially if you are stuck at home a lot, humans are social creatures.

Support Worksheet

Who can I talk to?

What's my plan for harder days?

Where can I go for support/information?

What I do:
Morning Stiffness

M orning stiffness is a characteristic symptom of Fibromyalgia, arthritis and rheumatism. An article on *Fibromyalgia Symptoms* website, *Morning Stiffness and Fibromyalgia* (n.d.), suggests that up to 90% of those with Fibromyalgia suffer from morning stiffness.

Morning stiffness means exactly what it sounds like: waking with stiff, aching muscles, usually the neck and spine. It can last an hour or linger for much of the day.

My neck and spine usually stiffen up over the course of the night. Movement returns slowly, over the morning. I am incapable of doing Pilates before lunchtime, my back will not co-operate, and it's usually as stiff as a board.

The National Fibromyalgia and Chronic Pain Association website has an article *10 Tips to Relieve Morning Stiffness* (n.d.) by Roger Chu, PhD, LAc, QME, and this list includes some basic ideas such as exercise, get enough sleep (easier said than done!), don't get too cold, eat healthier and deal with stress. I dislike weight, food and exercise as the big three ways to address everything in Fibromyalgia – I have eaten fairly healthily, kept to a healthy weight range and exercised beyond the minimum requirements since long before I was diagnosed. These are great whole of life tips, but they aren't going to magically cure things like morning stiffness.

Five Ways I Cope with Morning Stiffness

Low Dose Naltrexone (LDN)

Prior to LDN, my neck would get progressively stiffer as the night continued, resulting in multiple pillow changes, medication, non-medicated warming rub or my heat pack. By 5am, my neck would be too stiff to stay lying down, but my body too exhausted to get up. Now, I can get through the night on one pillow, rarely take medication, and sometimes don't need to use a non-medicated warming rub (Deep Heat).

Heat

Using my heat pack in the evening, taking it to bed to begin the night and applying it first thing in the morning are key for managing my neck. This requires almost 24/7 management. Heat is king. I set my children up with toast first thing so that I can sit with my heat pack and coffee. If I don't sit long enough my neck will remain stiff, tight and sore all day. If you have time, a warm shower can be useful also.

Stretching

Stretching, more specifically yoga poses help get my spine moving. Seated cat/cow pose, chair sun salutations, half sun salutations or full sun salutations really help get my body moving. These are easily found in a Google search.

Deep Heat/Heated Rub

When I can no longer sit still with my heat pack, I'll rub on this (it has a strong smell, so it's not ideal, but it does help).

Slowly Get Going

I rarely take medicine prior to 10am as I find once the fatigue and first stiffness ease, I tend to feel better. So I'll give my body some time to adjust to the day. If I had the time, a gentle walk would be ideal, but I'm usually rushing tiny ones out the door. And, actually, there isn't much medicine that would help anyway. My neck can occasionally be released by ibuprofen, spasms can be aided by a muscle relaxant, and headaches can sometimes be eased by paracetamol. Due to the low chances of these working I try to avoid them for as long as possible.

Morning stiffness is a common symptom, but there are plenty of things we can do to combat it.

10 Nice Minutes

I'm a fan of having a moment of nice in an otherwise tough day. If I'm lucky, my moment of nice is usually a good espresso that jolt only caffeine can give me that lasts a fleeting 10 minutes.

I've had a liberating thought. What if we reclaim our day? What if we add as many "10 Nice Minutes" as we possibly can?

Here's a list of the things we could do in 10 good minutes:

- Read (book nerd alert: always number one if my brain is not super fogged)
- Meditate
- Have a cup of tea or coffee and savour it
- A hot shower
- Lie down with a heat pack
- Lie down with a heat pack and a book
- Skype a dear friend or sister
- Eat a cupcake, or other deliciously good piece of food, savour it!

- Lie down with your legs up on a couch (yoga pose for calm)
- Watch half of a funny sitcom – or the whole thing and make it 20 good minutes!
- Sit in the sun
- Sit in the sun with a book
- Pray The Serenity Prayer with sincerity and meaning
- Read some good, inspiring blog posts that you've saved somewhere (like Pocket or Evernote)
- Give yourself a good foot rub
- Give yourself a good neck and shoulder massage with a heating cream
- Stretch, gently and mindfully
- Read a beautiful poem and just soak it up (I love Desiderata)
- Have a snuggle with your dog/cat/fluffy creature
- Have snuggles with your baby, if you have one and they let you!
- Some form of intimacy with your significant other (hug, kiss, nookie – hopefully that's more than 10 minutes)

- Breathe, deeply and mindfully
- Make your art (journal, write, colour, draw, imagine...)
- Write a "thankful list" for future reference

As you can see, for me, a lot of things revolve around reading, but that's because it's a big passion of mine. I encourage you to make a list of favourites for days when you need a reminder.

What I do: Work

Working is important to me. I worked hard to get to where I am in my career, despite working part-time for the past several years. It is also crucial for our financial well-being. Living is expensive, and coping with these illnesses is costly. Especially when it is more expensive to go the natural route than it is the medicine route.

Part-time work isn't always valued as highly as it should be. I have had to really convince some potential employers my value, despite only being available part-time. But there are some employers out there who get it, the value of a parent who has a decade of work experience and now is only available part-time. They have experience. They are typically more efficient, they tend to get in, do their work, and get out (back to their babies!). An area where advocacy is sorely needed is for those with chronic illnesses in the workforce.

I have found that if you don't give in, the right thing comes along. But you do have to really advocate for yourself. It's a gamble as to when and how you reveal your illnesses. I feel pretty sure I have been screened out for it, despite it being technically illegal. I have had precisely three understanding bosses, one of whom managed to follow through on their word to manage my workflow in such a way as to limit the stress on me. It's a work in progress and really depends on the person.

Trying not to get suckered into the prestige of high flying roles is difficult when your dream lies in living as well as you can with constant pain and fatigue. Trying to find the right role with the right hours so that you are not sacrificing too much of your precious energy away from your family is hard.

There's much I could say about work. But below I write some tips for managing brain fog at work and how working from home can benefit those with chronic illness.

Brain Fog at Work

Starting a new job is both a time of increased fatigue and an opportunity to begin good habits for managing yourself.

The first few weeks in a new job are always tiring. The brain fog then creeps in – losing words, muddling things up, and just plain forgetting things.

Luckily, there are a few ways to work with this:

Plan

I make sure I have a master list of the key projects, a date schedule for key tasks/deadlines and a daily to-do list. I work off this through the day and spend 10 minutes before I leave writing the next day's to-do list.

Prioritise

Choose what must be done immediately and what can wait. If it's early in the role and you aren't sure, ask the boss.

Rest

This is a hard one with children. The morning is rushed and there isn't much time for an afternoon rest. When there is a gap for a rest, take it. I have been known to park on the side of the road outside my children's carer's house, recline the seat and do a ten-minute meditation. If your partner/ support person is around in the afternoon or evening, take the opportunity to run off for a bath or shower – I like to do this early as I have no steam left once the children are down.

Sleep

Sleep is a generally problem for people with chronic illness, and it is a big struggle for me. If I'm lucky, I can spend about nine hours in bed and achieve eight hours of sleep. I try to get to bed by 9.30pm as often as I can to maximise sleep opportunity.

Exercise

It can slip when you're exhausted, learning a new routine and/or it's cold. However, even a 15-minute walk is counted as success for me. Keep it manageable and positive. Build yourself up for what you do; don't beat yourself up for what you don't.

Working From Home For Chronic Illness Fighters

Energy conservation and the ability to administer self-care are two very important elements of living well with chronic illness. Working from home, while a little isolating, is a great opportunity for chronic illness fighters. When I was contracting, it was also a fantastic way to be flexible around my husband and baby.

When I first went part-time, I also reduced my commute from an hour each way on the bus to 30 minutes in my car. This can save a lot of energy on its own. When I was working after I had Noah, I still had to drive him to and from his carer's place, but at least I didn't have to fight my way into town afterwards.

Here's my five top reasons why it's good to work from home:

1. You can administer your heat pack without looking like a granny.

2. You can use your breaks to lie down and pace the day as you need. (Eating is easier too – I'm a grazer, so

rather than eat a big lunch, I break it down into smaller meals.)

3. You can do yoga stretches without poking your butt out or getting on all fours in the office. And stretch your neck a lot without looking odd.

4. You have more control over your working area – temperature control, lighting, windows, etc. My home desk is set up perfectly for me and I have my Swiss ball if I get sick of my chair (this was basically the only way I could sit down for any length of time in the third trimester of all pregnancies – the back pain was unbelievable. Swiss balls are great).

5. You get heaps done without constant interruptions and without the little stressors the office provides. (Research suggests it takes something like half an hour to settle back into a task with each interruption.)

The Black Dog: Managing Emotions with Chronic Illness

In my travels through the research around Fibromyalgia and CFS, I keep coming across references to depression. Some doctors will try to say that Fibromyalgia is really depression.

I do have to confess that I do work hard to stay away from the "black dog." It is really hard to stay positive in the face of continual pain and (soul crushing) fatigue: think Groundhog Day with the flu.

There's no way to describe what it's like living with this. Or feeling like I'm continually letting down my husband and children. Or feeling trapped by the choices around work: balancing child care, losing a third of my income for someone else to look after my children, my neck, work opportunities, money. This one is a biggie for me.

I get sad. I feel angry.

The only person who suffers when I do too much is me. The increase in pain and fatigue is hard to take when it's already hard.

The balance is difficult.

A few tips for dealing with it include do the things that make you happy and do the amount of exercise you can and the type of exercise you enjoy.

Other things include:

- I enjoy my family – I get so many kisses and hugs daily, and I highly recommend this.

- Focus on the positive – write a list of your favourite things, the things you're thankful for and make the most of them.

- Journal – I write through everything. I find I can get a bit anxious or put stressful things on replay mode in my head. Writing it out can help.

- Have a bath with a book – this is my go-to relaxation choice and I do it often. I'll negotiate with my husband, he can nap and I'll have a bath. Find a little relaxation ritual that you could do daily.

- Talk to someone – I have my husband, my sister, Dana, and my brother, Luke. But if you don't have a person (especially one who gets the chronic illness), ask your doctor for options. I always find it cathartic to relay the symptoms I've been dealing with to my physio; they hear and they get it when they feel how tight or sensitive your muscles are!

- Know it's not a failure if you need an antidepressant – You deal with so much. You are amazing and this is because you know what you need to do to be well (whatever that means for you).

- Thank God – or the universe, or whatever you believe in, for the good things – there are so many good things.

Also know that, with the kinds of symptoms we are dealing with, it is reasonable to struggle with emotions. Of course we are sad when we are continually sore or miss out on fun things. Of course we are happy when we feel well.

It is wholly reasonable to grieve. And grieving with a chronic illness is not linear. Just when you think you have a handle on it, something will bring it all up again. And it's okay. If you're focusing relentlessly on how sad you feel, or lose the will to fight or just feel generally quite bad, then please seek help. You don't have to face it alone. You don't have to feel miserable.

And always know you are not alone. There are millions of us doing the fight together. Connect. Find fellow chronic illness fighters on Facebook, or in a local meet up.

Parenthood
With Chronic Illness

This is no small feat to have birthed and cared for three small children. It wasn't easy. But I don't regret it one bit. You will note the frequent mention of doing the fight with the children, because that is my context. They are so part of my life that all of my coping mechanisms must fit around them. But for this section, I'll focus specifically on doing parenting with a chronic illness. Generally, I am referring to my experience as a mama. But I hope this helps all parents, ones who have the baby physically or not.

Pregnancy

I am so passionate about sharing information about pregnancy and Fibromyalgia that I wrote a book about it. It was an eye opening experience to do pregnancy with these illnesses. When I had Noah, there was so little information; it just wasn't a nice experience. When I had Wyatt, there was a little more literature, and I had all of my knowledge, hard gained from my first experience. By the time I had Nathaniel, in 2018, I not only had my experience and research but I had a fantastic group of women in my Facebook group Pregnancy and Fibromyalgia to share the journey with – please do come and join if you are pregnant or intending to be!

Here are some of my key tips for being pregnant with chronic illness:

- Arm yourself with knowledge
- Get your body into the best place possible before conceiving
- Prioritise rest and sleep
- Nourish your body with good food and appropriate supplements
- Make a plan for the final trimester, delivery and the first six weeks that involves a good support system
- Get a pain management plan in place, discuss with your doctors what medicines you cannot come off, what you can and get your natural pain management mechanisms in place

Research shows that my experience will not dictate how you experience pregnancy. I found it far more difficult. Some actually experience a holiday from their symptoms. While it is useful to hear other people's experiences, so you don't feel like you're flying blind. The above six tips are the key things you need to know.

I had two crazy labour stories and then a fairly normal one. The first was posterior; he was backwards which caused severe back pain for the entire 20 hours. The second had the cord tied around him three times (unusual), and it was 52 hours (over both) of misery, but it was misery with an end date and the best pay off. My third gave me two days of pre labour and then just a few hours of active labour with only 24 minutes of pushing. It was intense! I can't tell if the Fibromyalgia made my experience of the pain worse

The one thing that seems to be more common is a flare up after the birth. The sleep deprivation, the pain, the 24/7 job that is looking after a baby are all rough. Get support. Choose your best support person and use them.

You can read about my nursing post on my blog or in my book, but here's what I will reiterate:

You count. You are absolutely part of this equation. If nursing hurts too much, if you hate it, if it's not working – you have the right to say no. Your baby needs you more than your boobs. (Yes breastmilk is nutritious and excellent, but not at the expense of the parent.)

It's not all or nothing. You can feed direct, express, top up with formula or all three. I lasted much longer with my second baby because I utilised all three of these options and it was a much better early parenting experience. With my third I was thankful to exclusively breastfeed past three months.

One day, one week, one month, one year – it's all success. Go you.

I will believe in each and every one of these points for the rest of my life. I will never allow a person to contradict these without a firm response. (Support people supporting new parents, please have their back here.)

Fourth Trimester

After the work of pregnancy, labour and the first few days, the most beautiful thing you can do for your baby and your body is to rest.

In places like India and Asia, women have a "lie in." For a month, they stay in bed and focus only on baby.

A Fourth Trimester to ease you and baby into life.

First and foremost, we need to be more caring towards ourselves. Pregnancy is a difficult time for even the healthiest women. Labour is hard. Adjusting to a tiny needy baby is a real test of endurance. So taking that time and not considering it business as usual is really important.

Particularly when you have a chronic illness for which pain and fatigue are already an issue. You're likely to flare up post birth. Sleep deprivation is no friend to pain or fatigue.

In order to give us a fair chance at succeeding in the endurance race that is the first year of having a new baby, let's consider the first few weeks as necessary resting/adjusting/healing time.

Some Useful Tips
for the Post-Birth Period

- Consider day and night as feasible sleeping times – try to arrange it so that you're not reliant on medicines that stop you getting to sleep without them. You may like to distinguish between night and day for baby: daytime feedings in the light, talking and singing, night-time feedings in dimmer light and more quiet.
- Sip on bone broth/soup broth for extra nutrients.

- Eat as best you can, despite potentially being too tired and sore to feel hungry. Consider smoothies with fruit and vegetables.
- Stay hydrated.
- Pelvic floor exercises!
- Let dad/partner/parent/friend take baby so you can rest and shower and eat and just be.
- Consider meditation for a nice booster (I love a guided meditation style called Yoga Nidra – 20 minutes is worth a few hours of sleep – and you can save varying lengths to your phone. Prayer is also meditative.)
- If you're breastfeeding, be wary of posture, hydration and fuel – it takes more energy than you may have.
- If you feel breastfeeding is a kick in the pants after your previous ordeals, as I did with Noah (far too painful and exhausting), don't feel guilty. You need to look after this baby and you for a long time yet, try to sense how much you can cope with before meltdown. Know that whatever you can give is beneficial. There are multiple options available to you.
- Switch between a comfortable chair/couch and your bed so your body doesn't get too sore from the same position.

- Jot down notes for your memory – I took many photos, videos and notes that I love looking back at.

- Store up some movies or TV series you might like to watch on some lazy days or when you're feeding.

- Have any supplements/medicines that you couldn't have while pregnant (and can have if breastfeeding) on hand, so that they're ready for you.

- Don't be too impatient to wean yourself off pain killers too fast. I forced myself off too soon with Noah thinking it was better to be less reliant on medicine, but I was only denying myself perfectly acceptable coping mechanisms.

Tricky Parenting Secret

Do you want to know a tricky wee parenting secret? It took a while to dawn on me. It doesn't take as much as you think to make a nice day for your kids.

Take a day in 2017 as an example: I was exhausted and my pain levels had been creeping up thanks to the baby waking up, up to six times a night. We went to church (with a baby and a three-year-old; it's not so peaceful anymore) and got frustrated with Noah not being quiet. We're not crazy –

we know he can't sit quietly for just over an hour. But not yelling would be great.

Back at home, he was frustrating us – we were feeling cabin fever but also the weight of the incomplete housework (sorry, our bathroom gets cleaned fortnightly now, eek). Baby wasn't playing ball with the napping. I was so tired I felt sick.

But we decided to go out. I wanted to be tired and sore out, instead of tired and sore at home. So we bundled into the car, drove half an hour, of which the baby slept 25 minutes (he was a chronic catnapper until five months), and visited a nice beach with a park. Parking was difficult, we got a 30-minute park, unbundled and faced the cold but beautiful scene. Noah happily rode his scooter up and down the beach, baby watched. On the way home, we stopped for chocolate sundaes at a special chocolate cafe.

Noah was difficult to keep occupied as we waited for our order. He was loud on the drive home.

But at the end of the day, as I remembered how frustrating it was to wrangle Noah and the overtired baby and my own issues. While admitting I had a nice time. Noah remembered a great day. He had fun. He remembered the scooter, the birds, the swing, and the chocolate sundaes. And our photos look so great.

All it took was a park and a treat. And I managed to give that to him (granted, with Husband's help), despite pain levels of 5/10 and fatigue levels up the whop.

It was a timely reminder as I worried about my lack of energy and time. As I worried that I didn't have enough to split between two kids.

But I do. I continually find reserves I didn't know I had, for their sakes. And my little efforts to keep Noah occupied pay off.

On days where we are housebound by baby and pain levels, Noah is just as happy to bake (he loves to stir) and colour, and ride his digger (as long as I'm watching) and snuggle while watching a movie.

So now my definition of a successful day is when I ask Noah, "Did you have a nice day?" And he responds with an emphatic "Yes!"

Parenting Resources

My book *Pregnancy and Fibromyalgia*

Pregnancy and Fibromyalgia Facebook group (I run this)

Fibro Parenting Facebook Group

Being Fibro Mom website

4 Lessons I have Learnt While Living With Fibromyalgia

After more than a decade fighting my Fibromyalgia, I couldn't imagine that the last two years could bring as much learning as it has. And this learning has produced four lessons.

Lesson One

Don't be surprised, or discouraged, if one avenue of potential healing doesn't produce results. A large school of thought in the cause of Fibromyalgia is that it is caused by underlying issues that need to be resolved. For example, thyroid issues, Candida, viral infections, allergies, etc.

Many Fibromyalgia bloggers/writers/doctors blame Candida overload for Fibromyalgia problems. They recommend cutting dairy and sugar and gluten and taking varying supplements. There are entire articles devoted to clearing

Candida. When I found out I had zero Candida in my system, I experienced a flare in my neck and fatigue.

I also have "optimal" results in the usual blood tests (thyroid, iron, antibodies, etc.). All worth checking and noting that "normal" does not always mean "optimal."

I don't give up, I store this in my "don't worry about it" column and move on.

Lessons Two & Three

Fibromyalgia is a massive undertaking of trial and error, which feeds into Lesson Three: you have to do the work yourself.

I have had precisely one doctor who is willing to listen to me, work with me and trial things with me in the 15-plus years I've been dealing with chronic pain. That doctor still doesn't have a lot of avenues to offer me, but he is willing to let me trial things I research. When I turned up with research papers prepared to be persuasive about a trial of low-dose Naltrexone, he agreed immediately.

I have tried a multitude of things to fight Fibromyalgia: physical therapies, like osteopathy, chiropractic, massage and physiotherapy (neck traction and acupuncture needles in trigger points help me); supplements, like MSM, magnesium, multivitamins, iron, olive leaf extract, probiotics and a truckload more I can't remember. (A helpful note here: using powders dissolved in water seems to absorb better than tablets for me).

Yoga, walking, stretching and swimming are helpful exercises that I enjoy. I have to modify for my neck and knees though. There's also a clearly defined line that I must keep to, and 25 mins of walking is enough; less causes pain in the lower body and more causes pain also.

Avoiding allergenic foods specific to me (bananas and dairy are occasional foods, corn and wheat are once per day foods according to my test). This was the one good thing that came out of hundreds of dollars spent on a naturopath. I trailed gluten-free eating a couple of years ago and found no effects while off or adding them back in. However, I do prefer non-glutinous grains like quinoa and millet as they have extra nutrients too.

There is a mind-body component. Meditation simultaneously helps me rest (I cannot nap) and teaches my central nervous system to calm down. Gratitude practice keeps me looking for the silver lining. Prayer helps sustain my hope (and hope is crucial, without that I'm done for). Colouring is calming and enjoyable. Reading is my favourite hobby and doesn't require physical activity. You need hobbies and you have a right to enjoy these even with a limited energy envelope.

Almost every time I read a book written by a Fibromyalgia doctor, I have found that I have made my way to an approximation of their protocols myself.

This is all by time consuming, expensive, roller coaster of emotions, trial and error.

Lesson Four

You can do *all* the things and still have Fibromyalgia.

Clearly, I do a lot to manage my health as best as I can. I have learnt a lot and do a lot, daily. But I still struggle everyday with these symptoms. Mostly my neck, fatigue and sleep.

I have come a long way since I was struggling through the day, so sore I wondered how my body was functioning, so exhausted I was nauseas most of the day and only managed by holding on to the glimmer of hope that getting enough work experience would mean I could earn enough per hour to reduce my work hours. But there is more to go until I am healed and I fight on.

How to Choose
A Treatment Option

Given the fact that there is no one answer for those of us with Fibromyalgia, no magic pill and no set treatment plan, we must find our own way. This is what this whole book is about: my own way.

So how should you assess treatment options?

Research

Check medicines and supplements on Drugs.com website.

Look for anecdotal evidence in the form of people with your symptoms or condition who also utilise that option. *Patients Like Me* and *Syndio* is a good website for tracking your health and treatments and accessing other's assessments of treatments.

Ask someone knowledgeable that you trust. Hopefully, you have at least one doctor in your corner for this.

Check for any interactions and side effects.

Checks it's safety in pregnancy if there's a chance you'll become pregnant in the near future.

Cost vs Benefit Assessment

Ask yourself:

Is the intended outcome worth the monetary investment? Is the intended outcome worth the potential side effects? What are the chances of the potential side effects affecting me?

What's the chance of success? What's the chance of failure? How much might it impact your life? What would happen as a result of it working?

Would you always wonder about it?

Plan

Plan for coping with potential side effects. Plan for administering the treatment option.

Document Your Experiment

This is crucial to assessing the impact. For example, the effects of low dose naltrexone took more than six months to manifest for me. It was subtle at first – I might have missed it if I weren't documenting my symptoms. Sometimes you have to stop a treatment to know for sure it was working – document this also.

Whole of Life Change: How it Looks Now

Please don't imagine my life is perfect, or that I am pain free. I'm not pedaling a cure. But I am in a much better place by following the things I have written about in this book. It is a journey I will be walking for my entire life.

My journey truly began when I trusted my instinct that life would be better if I reduced my work hours and cut the commute (an hour each way would diminish most people's energy levels).

I have learnt compassion, empathy, balance, gratitude, kindness and passion.

A lot of things have changed for me: I hardly ever lose words anymore, my memory is improving and so is my spacial awareness. The nausea is far less frequent and headaches only tend to bother me rarely– and they don't drive me to bed very often. My neck still causes me trouble, but the extreme tightness, dizziness, nausea and faintness is much rarer. My fight or flight response has calmed dramatically since I started meditating, which means I no longer overreact to scary stimulus and I don't panic as easily over things that used to make me anxious.

Most importantly, I am living life, not just coping.

I have a larger capacity for empathy. I have been forced to work only enough to live, with little stress, and I love it. Seeing friends bust their guts working 40-50 hours per week in jobs they don't love makes me thankful that I have learnt that I don't need the money or the prestige. I've gladly skipped the year living in London, buying fancy cars and clothes – because my dreams lie elsewhere.

My dreams lie in enjoying these amazing boys my husband and I made, in reveling in the fact that I get to be married to this man, and hopefully, in helping others learn to live well despite their circumstances.

I hope I make a difference in the lives of those that intersect with mine. I hope I always know what's important. I hope I always fight for my right to be well.

Resources: Facebook Groups, Books, Websites, Articles

- *Drugs.com* website
- *Deep-heat.co.uk* website
- *What Works For Fibromyalgia* Facebook Group
- *LDN Got Endorphins (Low Dose Naltrexone)* Facebook Group
- *Fibromyalgia and Muscle Pain: Your Guide to Self-Treatment* (2015) by Leon Chaitow ND, DO (book)
- *From Fatigued to Fantastic!* (2007) Jacob Teitelbaum, MD (book)
- *The FibroManual: A Complete Treatment Guide for You and Your Doctor* (2016) by Ginevra Liptan, MD (book)
- *Suffered Long Enough: A Physician's Journey of Overcoming Fibromyalgia, Chronic Fatigue and Lyme* (2014) by William Rawls, MD (book)
- *The Fibro Fix: Get to the Root of Your Fibromyalgia and Start Reversing Your Chronic Pain and Fatigue in 21 Days* by Dr David Brady
- *Fed up With Fatigue* website
- *Being Fibro Mom* website
- *ProHealth* website

- *LDN Research Trust* website
- *History of Fibromyalgia* (2013) by Dr Ananya Mandal, MD (article)
- *What is Fibro Fog? - Fibromyalgia and Cognitive Dysfunction* (2013) by Dr Ananya Mandal, MD (article)
- *11 Ways to Beat Fibro Fog* (2012) by Beth W. Orenstein (article)
- *Syndio Health* (website) (www.syndiohealth.com)

Acknowledgements

I was so pleasantly surprised by the amount of support my people gave me when I announced I had written my first book, *Pregnancy and Fibromyalgia*. Thank you to those who gave me encouraging words and those who bought that book. It gave me the courage to write this one, the one on my heart to share everything I have learnt, hoping it would help at least one person in their journey.

And thank you to these people:

Angela, for sending me the article that started my journey to wellness.

My parents for teaching me that no matter what difficulties we face, I am loved.

Lukie, for your tireless hours of editing, formatting and designing. This book *would not* have been completed were it not for you.

Dana, for being my favourite and the person I look up to. You and your wee family inspire me.

My husband and my children, Noah, Wyatt, and Nathaniel – the lights of my life, the loves of my life, the reasons I fight. This, and everything I do, is for you. Thank you.

God. My faith was the only thing that kept me putting one foot in front of the other as a young woman suffering severe pain and fatigue with no one to understand. Without that, I doubt I'd be here now.

About the Author

Melissa Reynolds has fought Fibromyalgia since she was 14 years old. Only, she didn't receive a name for her invisible opponent until she was in her 20s. Unfortunately, the name of the illness did not come with help.

After declaring war, she went from miserable and barely coping with life to thriving in seven years. Using a combination of research and personal trial and error, she has managed to bring her pain and fatigue levels down and minimise the effects of the debilitating brain fog by using everything she has written about on her blog.

This is Melissa's second book; her first book *Pregnancy and Fibromyalgia* was written to help parents with Fibromyalgia navigate pregnancy and nursing.

Melissa lives in Auckland, New Zealand, with her husband, three children, and her dog, Coop.

Before You Go

I hope this book has helped you. If you want to connect with me, you can find me:

- My blog: melissavsfibromyalgia.com (check out the Melissa vs Fibromyalgia Book page for free templates from this book);
- My Facebook: @confessionsofafibromama.

And could I ask you a favour? Could you please put a review on Amazon and Goodreads? Your review will help others who need information about fighting Fibromyalgia find it.

References

What is Fibromyalgia, Chronic Fatigue Syndrome and Myofascial Pain Syndrome?

Steven D. Ehrlich, NMD. (2016). *Fibromyalgia*. University of Maryland Medical Center. Retrieved from http://www.umm.edu/health/medical/altmed/condition/fibromyalgia

Sue. (2016). *Why Diagnosing Fibromyalgia Takes So Long*. FibroDaze. Retrieved from https://www.fibrodaze.com/diagnosing-fibromyalgia/

Adrienne Dellwo. (2017). *The History of Fibromyalgia*. Retrieved from https://www.verywell.com/the-history-of-fibromyalgia-716153

Dennis W. Dobritt, DO, DABPM, FIPP. *Fibromyalgia - A Brief Overview* (a presentation). Retrieved from https://www.michigan.gov/documents/mdch/fibroacpsm_246421_7.pdf

M.A. Fitzcharles & P. Boulos. 2003. Inaccuracy in the diagnosis of fibromyalgia syndrome: analysis of referrals. Retrieved from www.ncbi.nlm.nih.gov/pubmed/12595620

F Inanici, & MB Yunus. (2004). *History of Fibromyalgia: Past to Present*. PubMed. Retrieved from https://www.ncbi.nlm.nih.gov/pubmed/15361321

Dr Ananya Mandal, MD. (2013). *History of Fibromyalgia*. Retrieved from https://www.news-medical.net/health/History-of-Fibromyalgia.aspx

National Fibromyalgia & Chronic Pain Association. (n.d.). *Prevalence*. NFMCPA. Retrieved from https://www.fmcpaware.org/fibromyalgia/prevalence.html

Leonard A. Jason, Madison Sunnquist, Abigail Brown, Meredyth Evans, & Julia L. Newton. (2014). *Are Myalgic Encephalomyelitis and Chronic Fatigue Syndrome Different Illness? A Preliminary analysis.* PMC. Retrieved from https://www.ncbi.nlm.nih.gov/pmc/articles/PMC4125561/

Dr John Klippel. (n.d.). *Chronic Fatigue Syndrome and Fibromyalgia.* Retrieved from http://www.arthritis.org/living-with-arthritis/tools-resources/expert-q-a/fibromyalgia-questions/chronic-fatigue-syndrome-fibromyalgia.php

Dr Jacob Teitelbaum, MD. (n.d.). *EndFatigue.* Retrieved from http://endfatigue.com

Dr Jacob Teitelbaum, MD. (2007). *From Fatigued to Fantastic.* New York, NY: Avery.

Mayo Clinic. (n.d.). *Myofascial Pain Syndrome.* Retrieved from https://www.mayoclinic.org/diseases-conditions/myofascial-pain-syndrome/symptoms-causes/syc-20375444

Physician says fibromyalgia misdiagnosis is rampant. 2017. Retrieved from https://fedupwithfatigue.com/fibromyalgia-misdiagnosis/

What It's Really Like To Live With Chronic Pain and Fatigue

Paul Ingraham. (2008; 2017). *Insomnia's Role in Chronic Pain.* Retrieved from https://www.painscience.com/articles/insomnia-until-it-hurts.php

Paul Ingraham. (2011; 2017). *Central Sensitization in Chronic Pain.* Retrieved from https://www.painscience.com/articles/central-sensitization.php

Healing Journey Continued

CFIDS & Fibromyalgia Self-Help. (n.d.). *CFS & Fibromyalgia Rating Scale.* CFIDS & Fibromyalgia Self-Help. Retrieved from http://www.cfidsselfhelp.org/cfs-fibromyalgia-rating-scale

Bruce Campbell. (n.d.). *Understanding Your Situation.* CFIDS & Fibromyalgia Self-Help. Retrieved from http://www.cfidsselfhelp.org/library/understanding-your-situation

What I Do: Sleep

Ginevra Liptan. (2016). The FibroManual: A complete Fibromyalgia Treatment Guide for You and Your Doctor. Ballantine Books

Dr Ginevra Liptan. (n.d.). The FibroManual: A Complete Fibromyalgia Treatment Guide for You and Your Doctor (about page). Retrieved from http://www.drliptan.com/book/

Casey Thaler. (n.d.). 8 Tips for Better, More Effective Sleep. Paleohacks. Retrieved from https://blog.paleohacks.com/how-to-sleep-better/

Talk About Sleep. (2016). Sleep Disorders. Retrieved from https://www.talkaboutsleep.com/sleep-disorders/

What I Do: Pacing and Boundaries

Anne Leppert. (n.d.). Controlling Symptoms Through Pacing. Retrieved from http://www.cfidsselfhelp.org/library/control_through_pacing

What I Do: Meditation

Elaine R. Ferguson. (2013). Superhealing: Engaging Your Mind, Body, and Spirit to Create Optimal Health and Well-Being. HCL.

L.A. Martínez-Martínez, T. Mora, A. Vargas, M. Fuentes-Iniestra, & M. Martínez-Lavin. (2014). *Sympathetic nervous system dysfunction in fibromyalgia, chronic fatigue syndrome, irritable bowel syndrome, and interstitial cystitis: a review of case-control studies.* Retrieved from https://www.ncbi.nlm.nih.gov/pubmed/24662556

What I Do: Yoga

OSHU. (2010). School of Medicine Research Indicates Yoga can Counteract Fibromyalgia. OSHU. Retrieved from https://news.ohsu.edu/2010/10/14/school-of-medicine-research-indicates-yoga-can-counteract-fibromyalgia

Mia Park. (2014). Restorative Yoga Pose: Legs on a Chair. Yoga International. Retrieved from https://yogainternational.com/article/view/restorative-yoga-pose-legs-on-a-chair

Health.com. (n.d.). Child's Pose (video). Retrieved from http://www.health.com/health/m/video/0,,20731411,00.html

Clint Paddison. (2015). 7 Restorative Yoga Poses for Balance of Body, Mind, Spirit. Rheumatoid Arthritis Program. Retrieved from https://www.paddisonprogram.com/7-restorative-yoga-poses-for-balance-of-body-mind-spirit/

Kelly McGonigal. (2013). Restorative Yoga for Chronic Pain. Yoga International. Retrieved from https://yogainternational.com/article/view/restorative-yoga-for-chronic-pain

Elaine Gavalas. (2013). 3 Yoga Nidra Health Benefits. Huffpost. Retrieved from https://www.huffingtonpost.com/elaine-gavalas/yoga-nidra_b_2812676.html

Daniel Scott. (2012). Mastering the Yogic Breath. Mind Body Green. Retrieved from http://www.mindbodygreen.com/0-6751/Mastering-the-Full-Yogic-Breath.html

What I Do: Gentle Exercise

W. Häuser, P. Klose, J. Langhorst, B. Moradi, M. Steinbach., M. Schiltenwolf, & A. Busch. (2010). Efficacy of different types of aerobic exercise in fibromyalgia syndrome: a systematic review and meta-analysis of randomised controlled trials. PubMed. Retrieved from https://www.ncbi.nlm.nih.gov/pubmed/20459730

Angela J. Busch, Sandra C. Webber, Mary Brachaniec, Julia Bidonde, Vanina Dal Bello-Haas, Adrienne D. Danyliw, Tom J. Overend, Rachel S. Richards, Anuradha Sawant, and Candice L. Schachter. (2011). Exercise Therapy for Fibromyalgia. Retrieved from https://www.ncbi.nlm.nih.gov/pmc/articles/PMC3165132/

What I Do: Physiotherapy and Acupuncture

John C Deare, Zhen Zheng, Charlie CL Xue, Jian Ping Liu, Jingsheng Shang, Sean W Scott, & Geoff Littlejohn. (2013). Acupuncture for treating fibromyalgia. Retrieved from https://www.ncbi.nlm.nih.gov/pmc/articles/PMC4105202/

Dr Diana Cross. (n.d.). Acupuncture & Pain. Retrieved from http://www.pain-education.com/trigger-points.html

What I Do: Medicine – Low Dose Naltrexone

Donna Gregory Burch. (2016). Low Dose Naltrexone – An Effective Treatment for ME/CFS? Retrieved from http://www.pro-health.com/library/showArticle.cfm?libid=28903&site=articles

Jarred Younger, Luke Parkitny, & David McLain. (2014). The Use of Low-Dose Naltrexone (LDN) as a Novel Anti-Inflammatory Treatment for Chronic Pain. PMC. Retrieved from https://www.ncbi.nlm.nih.gov/pmc/articles/PMC3962576/#!po=11.0390

UAB, College of Arts and Science. (n.d.) Current Projects. Retrieved from https://cas.uab.edu/

Dr Phil Boyle. (n.d.). Low Dose Naltrexone in Pregnancy. Retrieved from http://www.ldn2016.com/sites/default/files/Dr-Phil-Boyle.pdf

Drugs.com. (n.d.). Naltrexone Use While Breastfeeding. Retrieved from https://www.drugs.com/breastfeeding/naltrexone.html

What I do: Medicine – Amitriptyline

Leon Chaitow, ND, DO. (2015). Fibromyalgia and Muscle Pain: Your Guide to Self-Treatment. Conari Press.

What I do: Supplements

Dr Axe. (n.d.). 8 Natural Ways to Overcome Fibromyalgia Symptoms. Retrieved from https://draxe.com/fibromyalgia-symptoms/

Fibromyalgia Treatment Group. (n.d.). 10 Herbs and Supplements to Try for Fibromyalgia Pain. Retrieved from http://fibromyalgiatreatmentgroup.com/fibromyalgiatreatment/10-herbs-supplements-to-try-if-you-have-fibromyalgia

Sue. (2014). 14 Supplements That May Help Fibromyalgia. Retrieved from https://www.fibrodaze.com/14-supplements-help-fibromyalgia/

Dr Jacob Teitelbaum. (n.d.). Nutrition Guide. Retrieved from https://secure.endfatigue.com/nutrition-guide

Dr. Jacob Teitelbaum. (2013). The Fatigue and Fibromyalgia Solution. Avery.

EndFatigue. (n.d.). Book: The Fatigue and Fibromyalgia Solution. Retrieved from https://secure.endfatigue.com/store/products/publications/bkfafs/index.html

What I Do: Brain Fog

Arthritis Foundation. (n.d.). *Fibro Fog: Sleep, brain dysfunction likely culprits for cognitive difficulties associated with fibromyalgia*. Retrieved from http://www.arthritis.org/about-arthritis/types/fibromyalgia/articles/fibro-fog.php

What I Do: Food

Shannon Harvey. (2016). The Whole Health Life: How You Can Learn to Get Healthy, Find Balance and Live Better in The Crazy-Busy Modern World. Whole Health Life Publishing.

What I do: Morning Stiffness

Fibromyalgia Symptoms. (n.d.). Morning Stiffness and Fibromyalgia. Retrieved from https://www.fibromyalgia-symptoms.org/fibromyalgia_morning_stiffness.html

Roger Chu. (n.d.). 10 Tips to Overcome Morning Stiffness. Retrieved from https://www.fmcpaware.org/fundraising/176-movement-therapies/907-10-tips-to-overcome-morning-stiffness.html

Made in the USA
Monee, IL
02 September 2022